The Soul
of
Medicine

—Tales from the Bedside—

SHERWIN B. NULAND

KAPLAN PUBLISHING

New York

This publication is designed to provide accurate and authoritative information in regard to the subject matter covered. It is sold with the understanding that the publisher is not engaged in rendering legal, accounting, or other professional service. If legal advice or other expert assistance is required, the services of a competent professional should be sought.

© 2009 by Sherwin B. Nuland

Published by Kaplan Publishing, a division of Kaplan, Inc.
1 Liberty Plaza, 24th Floor
New York, NY 10006

Printed in the United States of America

10 9 8 7 6 5 4 3 2 1

Library of Congress Cataloging-in-Publication Data
Nuland, Sherwin B.
   The soul of medicine : tales from the bedside / by Sherwin B. Nuland
     p. ; cm.
   Includes bibliographical references and index.
   ISBN 978-1-60714-055-9 (alk. paper)
   1. Medicine--Anecdotes. I. Title.
   [DNLM: 1. Medicine--Personal Narratives. 2. Physicians--Personal
Narratives. WZ 112 N969s 2009]
   R705.N847 2009
   610--dc22
                                      2008048289

To Sarah, to Sal,

Always and ever, but especially now

CR

Contents

Prologue ix

The Surgeon's Tale 1

The Family Physician's Tale 17

The Dermatologist's Tale 31

The Gastroenterologist's Tale 35

The Obstetrician-Gynecologist's Tale 41

The Ophthalmologist's Tale 45

The Cardiologist's Tale 55

The Pediatric Cardiologist's Tale 65

The Anesthesiologist's Tale 73

The Neurosurgeon's Tale(s) 87

The Chest Surgeon's Tale(s) 101

The Medical Student's Tale 117

The Geriatrician's Tale(s) 123

The Bronchoscopist's Tale 135

The Internist's Tale 143

The Surgeon's Second Tale 155

The Nephrologist's Tale 161

The Neurologist's Tale(s) 175

The Urologist's Tale 183

The Pediatrician's Tale 193

The Narrator's Tale 197

Epilogue 205

Index 209

~

Prologue

L IKE ALL DOCTORS, I collect stories. Over my thirty years in the practice of surgery and afterward, I have heard many case narratives and personal recollections, and more than a few of them have stuck so fast in my mind that I can recall details just as they were told to me. Some of the stories are interesting for their own sake but go far beyond mere factual description to teach lessons. In certain ways, they are the lessons of humanity itself, with all its wondrous gifts and its failings. In others, the themes to be considered are unique to medicine, whether as a branch of science or an aspect of the relationship between individuals. Within the covers of this book lies—with only the faintest of apologies to Geoffrey Chaucer—a sort of *Canterbury Tales* of medicine.

Every transaction between doctor and patient is a transaction in personal and professional ethics. And it is also an exercise in confidentiality. The ethical obligations are sometimes obvious and other times obscure. For such reasons, I have in certain cases found it useful to add a commentary to a story, while I have chosen merely to tell the other tales as first-person narratives, in the way they were told to me. In this, I have tried to approximate the manner of the original storyteller, because I believe writing in that way adds to the immediacy of what is being read.

As for confidentiality, I have employed a simple and commonly used device—using the medical facts to reconstruct a series of events in which everything but those facts is so well disguised that the identity of patient, doctors, and other individuals is hidden. In doing this, I have changed far more than names. A tall man may appear here as short; a name of one ethnicity is usually changed to another; the director of a music collection may be put in charge of a rare book library; a patient may be given a university degree he never had. Some of the stories have required very little alteration and some far more. But the important thing about all of them is that the medical facts in the following pages are just as they happened. This is a book of nonfiction.

Writing in this way has allowed me to do certain other things that I had not anticipated at the outset. Because almost all of the physicians are men and women for whom I have long had high regard, it has given me the opportunity to demonstrate aspects of the ethics of medicine and the ways in which certain technological changes and patient advocacy groups have affected them or may affect them in the future. I describe that sacrosanct connection between two people that we call the doctor-patient relationship, and that other relationship, between mentor and student, so important to the perpetuation of medical knowledge, judgment, wisdom, and character. Doctors have particular ways of approaching certain kinds of problems, many of which have found their way into this book.

The Soul

of

Medicine

꙳

The Surgeon's Tale

S OMETIMES IT SEEMS THAT our most unusual cases are ones we see during those hectic years of residency. If I had to choose my own most bizarre experience on the ward, it would have to be my encounter with Jimmy Tyson and his chest full of pus.

I was resident on the chest service at the time, and just getting ready to make late rounds on a Friday evening when I heard myself being paged to one of the medical units, Raleigh I. When I got there with the intern, a fellow named Harry Clark, I was shown the chart and chest X-ray of a nineteen-year-old kid who had been admitted three days earlier with a fever of 103 and a complete white-out of the left side of his chest—it was totally opaque, even though the right side was perfectly clear and normal. The film and clinical course had all the earmarks of an empyema, but there was no history or any other clue to explain it. An empyema is a collection of pus that accumulates between the chest wall and the lung because the inner lining of the chest cavity is irritated, usually by some bacteria-laden substance. The lining, called the pleura, secretes or pours the fluid forth so that it forms a constricting pool around the lung. If there's enough of it, the lobes of the lung are compressed and breathing is compromised. The medical interns had been putting needles into young Tyson's chest over and over, hoping to drain out as much of the fluid as possible and allow the lung to expand properly, in addition to getting a sample of the pus in order to identify the offending bacteria. But every effort had been futile. In typical overly relaxed-and-then-sudden-panic medical-intern fashion, they'd waited until Friday evening to ask for a surgical consultation.

Without hiding my displeasure at being called so late, I tried to extract some of the pus by sticking a few big, wide-bore needles into the fellow's back and side at three or four different levels. When I started, I thought the problem was just the medical interns' inexperience, but with each stick I wondered more and more. Whatever this pus was, it seemed too thick for my widest-gauge needle. Even the kid's blood cultures had been negative, and the interns had finally started him on a broad-spectrum antibiotic in the hope of getting some control over his illness. I kept talking to the boy as I worked, not so much to distract him as to try to elicit some story that would explain his problem, but all he would tell me was that he'd started to feel lousy about four days earlier, gone to the emergency room, and here he was, getting sicker every day. It was becoming pretty obvious that this boy needed to go to the operating room. I planned to lay him on his right side and infiltrate some local anesthesia into a small area over one rib, remove about an inch of the bone, and open into his left chest to see what was there. I'd then insert a wide tube snugly into the thoracic cavity in order to drain at least some of the pus. That way we could get material for bacterial identification, gradually empty the pus, and allow the underlying compressed lung to expand.

Jimmy was a tough street kid from New Haven's black ghetto and swore constantly while we were taking him up to the OR, even though he'd been tight-lipped while needle after needle was being stuck into his chest, giving only the briefest of grunted answers to my questions. No family, no friends—I wasn't even sure whether the operative permit he'd grudgingly signed was legal. He'd murmured something that I'm pretty sure was "What the fuckin' hell—you'll do it anyway" when he handed the paper back to me. As you might expect, he accused each of us, individually and collectively, of having sex with our mothers.

In the OR, Harry and I injected lidocaine and I made a three-centimeter incision down to the bone. I loosened about an inch of rib from the surrounding tissue, clipped the bit of rib out, and then made an incision through the thickened underlying layer of pleura. And then came the surprise. It wasn't ordinary pus that came pouring out under pressure—the stuff was a light brown color and smelled like shit. Fact is, a couple of small bits of solid feces came out with it. I glanced over at Harry, whose eyes had widened over his mask as he looked at me for some sort of answer to the question he didn't need to ask—how does feces get into the chest of a nineteen-year-old kid who'd been perfectly healthy before this present episode?

It was obvious that I'd have to open the chest all the way, because some crazy thing had happened inside it. The standby anesthesiologist was as flummoxed as Harry and I were, but he explained very patiently to the kid that solving his problem would be more work than we'd anticipated, so he'd need a general anesthetic. Jimmy only nodded his head, swore a little more, and was asleep with a breathing tube down his throat in little more than a minute.

Then the surprises *really* began. Once I had the left side of the chest spread wide open, the suction bottle filled up with about two liters of this same thick, disgusting stuff, while Harry and I lifted out close to a handful of small pieces of stool. When we had the whole thoracic cavity cleaned and irrigated, we changed into fresh gowns and gloves, got a new set of sterile instruments, and took a good look inside.

The problem was obvious, and one glance downward at the diaphragm explained everything. The diaphragm is a thick sheet of muscle and fiber lying transversely across the middle of the body, separating the chest cavity from the abdomen. Its only openings are three snug apertures that allow the esophagus and the large artery and vein called the aorta and vena cava to traverse it; it is otherwise like an intact, inviolate curtain of flesh through which nothing can pass. That may describe your diaphragm or mine, but not the unique one possessed by Jimmy Tyson. Jimmy's had an extra hole near its front, or anterior, part with which he'd obviously not been born. Through that hole, a bit of the upper edge of the transverse colon had somehow intruded itself from the abdomen below, gotten pinched off because the opening was so small, been strangulated, and then perforated into the thoracic cavity. All the havoc, all the junk in the chest, was the result of little bits of stool and feculent liquid from the bowel having emptied into the chest. What this boy had was essentially what you might call a shit empyema.

It was pretty clear what had to be done. The nurses readjusted the drapes, and we swabbed the belly with sterilizing solution. I made a short transverse incision in the left upper quadrant of the abdomen, coming down precisely on the place where the colon was stuck into the hole in the diaphragm. I put specialized clamps on each side of the involved intestine and cut loose the trapped knuckle of bowel from the herniated part clinging to the undersurface of the diaphragm. It was a simple matter to remove the bit of perforated colon and bring the healthy ends out through the short abdominal incision as a temporary transverse colostomy, which I'd be able to reconnect in about three weeks. We changed gloves and turned our attention back to the chest. The hole in the diaphragm was so small that it took no more than my pinky to fill it. I repaired it with a few carefully placed sutures, closed the chest, and stepped back to think, when the kid woke up, screaming and thrashing his arms wildly in every direction.

How had the hole gotten there? It looked nothing like the congenital diaphragmatic hernias that are on rare occasions found in infants; in fact, it had the appearance of having been man-made, perhaps with a sharp instrument like a narrow-bladed knife. The patient's past hospital record consisted of only a single emergency room sheet from a visit four years earlier, and the medical intern had told me during my consultation that there was no point in my reading it because the scrawled note on its front couldn't possibly provide any clues to the presence of an empyema. I figuratively kicked my own ass for not having looked at it, then went downstairs to the medical floor as fast as I could, where the emergency room sheet still lay in its folder amid a pile of old patient charts.

And there it was—the answer to the feculent puzzle. At fifteen, Tyson had come into the emergency room with a very short slash through the skin just under his left rib cage, no greater than two centimeters in length and appearing to have barely penetrated the fatty layer underneath—or so it was described in the brief emergency room note. Because it seemed not only minor but superficial, the intern on duty had dressed it with antibiotic gauze and told the boy to return to the surgical clinic in three days, which he never did.

If that piece of information made me feel stupid, going back up to the recovery room to inspect the patient's abdomen only worsened the anguish. In paying so much attention to Jimmy's chest, I had neglected to look carefully at anything else. But now with a bright light focused on it, I could see the old wound clearly—thin as a razor blade and shrunken to half its original length, staring up at me from its easily visible hiding place just under the left rib margin. The boy was by then wide awake, and I asked him how he had gotten the tiny scar. The answer was brief and to the point: "Motherfucker stuck a knife in my belly when I wouldn't give him my Red Sox jacket. Could'a cut me in my heart, the prick." On further questioning it turned out that "motherfucker" had plunged the blade upward as far as the handle, probably realized what he'd done, then pulled the knife out and taken off in a panic. When the small wound healed uneventfully, Jimmy thought everything was fine. He had no idea that he was now the possessor of a brand-new hole in his diaphragm, which would never heal itself closed as his skin had done. He had not had any problems until less than a week before he came into the hospital, when he developed episodes of colicky pain in the evening after eating supper. The feverishness and shortness of breath began a few days later.

Everything added up. The tip of the blade had indeed made a permanent hole in the left side of Jimmy's diaphragm. About a week before the present episode, a bit of transverse colon had snaked its way through the hole—I have no idea why it took four years to make up its mind to commit such mischief—and gotten pinched off, lost its blood supply, and perforated into the chest, with all the foul consequences we discovered at operation. I had never heard of such a thing; in fact, during the thirty years I practiced surgery after that eventful night, I never saw or heard of anything remotely resembling it. But there was another surprise yet to come.

I looked up at the big clock on the wall of the recovery room and saw that it was already almost 3:00 A.M., which meant that I'd have barely four hours of sleep before Surgical Grand Rounds, the weekly teaching conference attended by the entire staff. It also meant that it would be only a short time before I could tell my chief, Professor Swenson, about the fascinating patient I'd cared for and the way I had invented a solution for his problem, which I was by then considering quite skillful under the difficult circumstances of having encountered an entirely new medical entity. I rushed up to the on-call room but found myself too excited to get more than a few fitful and very brief lapses into sleep. Promptly at 7:30 I appeared at the door to the chief's office just as he was opening it in anticipation of my arrival, it being our custom to confer each morning at that time to discuss any new cases that had arrived since the previous day.

The chief was a dour, humorless Swede under the best of circumstances, and the early morning hours were his worst. So I was quite naturally surprised—and more than a bit disturbed—when I noticed that my enthusiastic recitation was causing what seemed to be the tiniest trace of a smile trying to make its appearance at the usually downturned corners of his mouth. He was about two inches shorter than I, and had two of the bushiest brows I've ever encountered. But even looking down through those hirsute brambles, I could see that his pale blue eyes were twinkling. He had a habit to which every one of his residents quickly became accustomed, which was to rock back and forth from the heels to the balls of his feet when he was about to deliver himself of some pithy statement—and this was precisely what he had begun to do. We used to call that movement "Swenson's foot sign," but its significance paled in comparison to "Swenson's stethoscope sign," which was reserved for the most meaningful of utterances, and this, too, had made its appearance. Like many chest surgeons of those days, the professor always wore the irons of his stethoscope clasped around his neck, ready to slip into his ears at a second's notice, and the "sign" consisted of his flipping back and forth the tubing from which the old-fashioned metal listening-bell hung. With both clues in a kind of harmonic motion with each other, I knew that my notions of discovery and triumph were in some danger, a feeling confirmed when, at the end of my peroration—I believe the final words were something like "Don't you think I should publish it as an original observation? Might even end up being called Nuland's syndrome"—he broke into the first broad smile I had ever seen on his face and said, very quietly, "I suppose you think you're the only surgeon ever to have seen such a thing." I was mumbling something meant to signify that he was right, when he turned on his heel and beckoned me to follow him into his office.

Professor Carl Gustaf Swenson was a widely read medical historian and a collector of antique books, all of which he kept on a high bank of shelves alongside his desk. Getting up on tiptoe, he pulled a huge old folio volume down from the top shelf and showed me the title, which required just about nothing of my high school French to translate as *The Works of Ambroise Paré*. The name of Paré was well known to me: he was a sixteenth-century French surgeon renowned not only for his innovations but for having written many books about the patients he treated on the battlefield and elsewhere, all in vernacular unlike the more learned physicians, who wrote Latin in a style comprehensible only to the well educated, which the surgeons of the time certainly were not.

Swenson laid the book carefully down on his desk and began gingerly to turn the pages with such a delicate surgeon's hand that only a few bits of browned edge separated themselves from the brittle paper. At last he found what he was looking for, and pointed to it as though he had just rediscovered the name of some obscure Norse town on an ancient map of Vinland. "There it is, Nuland—read it!" It took a while, but accepting his help with an occasional word, I finally made my way through the Renaissance French.

The patient Paré described was a certain Captain François d'Alon of Xantoigne, who was serving at the siege of La Rochelle in 1567 when he was hit near the cartilaginous extension of the breastbone by a musket ball that exited laterally between the left fifth and sixth ribs. The outer wound healed, but he continued to have episodes of colicky pain every evening after supper and through the night. At some point during the eighth month after the injury, the pain suddenly became worse and he died days later. At autopsy, a loop of transverse colon was found to have pushed its way into the chest through a hole in the diaphragm so small that it was—and to this day I remember the words as they stared up at me from the discolored and fragile page—*comme un petit doigt,* "like a little finger." In later years I would own the first English translation of the book, done in 1634, where the words were translated as "a wound of the diaphragm so small that you could scarce put your little finger in thereat." The captain had died of the disease I was prematurely calling Nuland's syndrome, but too quickly for an empyema to have developed. The professor closed the book, asked me to return it to the shelf, and then did a very uncharacteristic thing: He put his arm around my shoulders and together we walked into Grand Rounds, like father and son.

∝

Commentary to The Surgeon's Tale

Among the wonderful fascinations of practicing medicine is the continuing thread that runs through its entire millennia-long history. Science changes, but human nature does not. As long as one human being is called upon to treat another, bits of story will repeat themselves, similar dilemmas will be confronted, and repetition of seemingly new challenges will appear as though for the very first time.

In the Tale just narrated—which is my own—I stated that in years of searching, I have never come across another case like Jimmy Tyson's: "I never saw or heard of anything remotely resembling it." And yet, even while inscribing those words onto the lined paper on which I habitually write, I wondered about them—even wondered whether some medical reader would write to contradict me through his or her own experience. In this age of rapid computer searches, it should be possible to find a few reports of feculent empyema caused by an unrecognized traumatic hernia in the diaphragm, perhaps even of a size "*comme un petit doigt.*" I have found none, nor have any appeared in the anecdotal or historical literature I often read. And precisely what does such an absence mean? Probably nothing. Nothing, that is, except that any other observers encountering such cases, whether in the operating or autopsy room, have not recorded them. Or perhaps it speaks of my own inefficiency with computer technology. Is it really possible that Jimmy Tyson and Captain d'Alon are the only people whose diaphragms have been pierced by an instrument of war or anger, leaving a permanent opening into which a piece of gut eventually intruded itself? I doubt it.

Ambroise Paré was a prolific writer. He described every case he saw from which he believed something might be learned by his fellow surgeons; hundreds upon hundreds of patients are included in his collected works. In this, he was unique; no surgeon of his time or for centuries afterward did such a thing. Who knows what they might have written had they his relentless drive to record everything? And who knows how many surgeons of our time have been unwilling to put themselves through the editorial exertions nowadays required to publish a case report? And so, who knows how many Tysons and d'Alons there have actually been?

I am reminded here of the dramatic outpouring of acclaim when ether-induced sleep was introduced on an October morning in 1846, at the Massachusetts General Hospital. The day before, surgical anesthesia had not existed; during the following weeks, word of its efficacy was spreading throughout the world. The man who performed the first operation under anesthesia, Harvard's John Collins Warren, proclaimed with the voice of unimpeachable authority that "a new era has opened on the operating surgeon." In retrospect, Warren's certainty that he was the first to operate under ether had to have been a fantasy, as have so many other claims of priority or uniqueness.

Ether had been synthesized by a Prussian botanist named Valerius Cordus in 1540, and its soporific properties are known to have been recognized at least as early as the first years of the nineteenth century, when "ether frolics" became a common form of participatory entertainment among young bon vivants of the time. Everyone who went to such parties knew that a person inhaling enough of the volatile vapor fell into a deep sleep. Surely, there must have been a few surgeons in New York or Paris who took advantage of that effect to painlessly amputate an occasional leg or remove an unsightly cyst from a bald scalp. But such adventurous souls probably thought of ether as a simple aid in their work—though perhaps a daring one—and never stopped to consider the potentially stupendous implications of what they were doing. In fact, one of them, Crawford Long of Georgia, is known to have used ether to remove a cyst from the neck of one James Venable four years before Warren's feat. Had the Western world been canvassed in 1846, there is little doubt that hundreds of similar stories might have been repeated by a multitude of physicians, not a one of them having thought to write an article about what he had done.

So, statements like "I never saw or heard of anything remotely resembling it" should be taken with the grain of salt I'm now inserting into my narrative. It has only been since the mid-twentieth century that every eructation emerging from a laboratory or clinic is reported in the medical literature, lest priority be claimed by some other burper. As memorable as the case of Jimmy Tyson may have been, its uniqueness proved to be only in my mind.

I cannot leave this Tale and go on to the next without relating the story of how I came to own the 1634 translated edition of Paré's massive 1,200-page opus. It was presented to me by the widow of its previous owner, who had in turn been given it by the physician in whose possession it had been for several decades, and so forth all the way back to its original printing almost four hundred years ago. Neatly inscribed on a small sheet of blue paper tucked into the book's cover was a list of the names of every man who had owned it until the late eighteenth century. A gap then appears between that time and when "Thomas Andrews Jr. bought the book in 1846" as indicated by a written notation on the flyleaf. The names of three more recent owners appear after a space on the blue sheet, ending with my own. The custom of passing this book on to a physician who is also a historian will continue with my death. Though he does not know it, I have already chosen the recipient.

As for Jimmy Tyson: Following a stormy course of pneumonia and partial collapse of his left lung, he finally overcame every obstacle and recovered from his Friday night adventure in the operating room. After three weeks in a supervised convalescent facility, he returned to the hospital for reattachment of the separated parts of his transverse colon. Even that second procedure was not without complication, this one being a significant wound infection in the tissues of the abdominal wall near his newly approximated bowel. By the time everything healed, Jimmy had spent a total of more than three months in the hospital or under direct medical supervision at the convalescent facility.

I'd love to be able to report that Jimmy emerged from his ordeal a changed man. My fantasy would be that his realization of the many nurses and doctors who truly cared about him allowed qualities in his character to come forth that had been submerged by the difficult life he led before that auspicious night in the operating room.

The fantasy would go on to become a success story in which Jimmy found a job, acquired a high school equivalency diploma, and went on to a successful and useful life. And perhaps that is actually what happened. But the facts are probably otherwise. After one visit to the outpatient clinic, he never returned for his next appointment. None of us who cared for Jimmy Tyson ever saw him again.

The Family Physician's Tale

WE WERE TAUGHT NEVER to let ourselves fall in love with a patient, but no one ever said anything about a crush. Mine started the moment I laid eyes on her, and who could blame me? She was a tall, green-eyed, honey-haired blonde, with a figure like Esther Williams and a mind like Arlene Francis—remember them? I was a twenty-five-year-old third-year medical student just as short and dorky as I am today, and she talked to me as though I were Dr. Kildare, the handsome young intern played by Lew Ayres in so many movies. I couldn't believe my luck in being assigned to do her admission history

and physical exam, my very first day as a clinical clerk on the
General Surgery service in 1955.

Her problem was simple enough. She was a thirty-two-year-
old married woman with a three-centimeter nontender lump
in the side of her left breast. She had first become aware of it
about eighteen months earlier, but "I'm not one to go to doctors, so I didn't do anything until I developed this little infection
from shaving under my armpit, and noticed that a few glands
had gotten swollen. Thinking I'd need antibiotics, I went to see
Dr. Frei, who suggested I have the lump removed for biopsy as
soon as the infection cleared." She spoke in complete and very
literate sentences, which was hardly surprising because she was
an editor at the Canterbury Press and her husband was a well-
known political journalist, whose name you'd recognize if I said
it, even now more than fifty years later.

I heard these little bits of information while taking her clinical history, but the most important part didn't turn up until
later, while I was doing the physical exam. The rule was that
every woman had to have a pelvic, and it was usually done by the
medical student, supervised by an assistant resident. This served
a double purpose: to get it done and recorded, and to have the
assistant resident looking over the student's shoulder as a kind
of instructor, both to teach and to be sure everything was being
carried out correctly.

One of the nurses positioned the patient—whom I'll call
Arlene Williams, to combine my idealized notion of brains and
body—on an examining table and into stirrups, and I began the
exam by sliding two gloved, lubricated fingers into the vaginal

opening. But something that felt like a dense screen kept me from going any farther. I looked up over my right shoulder at the assistant resident— it was Joe Forkner, who later went into practice in Michigan City, Indiana—and motioned for him to take my place. After settling himself on the stool, he attempted the same maneuver, but I could see that he was being stopped too, and couldn't force his way through what felt like a thick sheet of tissue lying across the vaginal opening to obstruct the passage. He had the nurse shine a light on it and the puzzle was immediately, if surprisingly, solved: The obstacle was a perfectly normal though unusually thick and leathery hymen, with only a small perforation in its center, no bigger than a centimeter in diameter but otherwise completely intact. It was the kind of thing you'd expect in a virginal teenage girl, allowing menstrual flow to pass through but not much else.

We took Mrs. ("Ms." hadn't yet been invented) Williams down off the examining table, and all three of us sat ourselves in comfortable chairs in the empty visitors' lounge so that the obvious question could be asked in as un-awkward (is there such a word?) manner as possible. Yes, she told us; though she and her husband were deeply in love, they'd never been able to have sexual intercourse and just assumed this was how it had to be. In fact, they were in the early stages of adopting a baby. They'd reconciled themselves to Mrs. Williams having been born with some sort of anatomical abnormality, and, being the kind of private people they were, had not mentioned it to their family doctor. Consequently, she'd never seen a gynecologist and had no idea that opening what Joe now told her was an imperforate, abnormally thickened hymen was a simple procedure that could be done in minutes, while she was under anesthesia for the breast biopsy. Those strikingly lovely eyes glowed when she heard that she would then be able to have a normal sex life, and she broke out in a wide smile as she described her excitement at the thought of being able to tell her husband.

A story like the one I've been telling you is unimaginable nowadays, but this was during the mid-1950s, when so many people were very naïve about sex. Here was an attractive, well-educated young woman who'd been married seven years and had no idea that simple ignorance was keeping her from the kind of fulfillment for which every woman should have the opportunity. Joe said he'd inform Dr. Wallace, the operating surgeon, about the situation, and a gynecologist would see the patient later that afternoon and arrange to open the hymen. As we walked down the corridor together, Joe and I were marveling at the situation in which we had become involved, in which a consultation for a simple breast biopsy would change the lives of two people.

When Joe left, I went back, talked the whole thing over with Mrs. Williams, and asked her to sign the operative permit. This was my first experience at obtaining a permit, and it was one that bore the strangest mixture of procedures I would ever see. All breast biopsies in those days required hospital admission, and every permit called for the patient's consent that the surgeon could do a radical mastectomy should the biopsy prove to be positive, even when the chance was as remote as it was in the case of Mrs. Williams. And so, in the blank space on the form where the name of the operation was to be filled in, I wrote the following: "breast biopsy, radical mastectomy and hymenotomy," and that's the way it appeared when the operating room schedule was posted late that evening. I'll bet it raised plenty of eyebrows around the hospital.

Mrs. Williams—by then we were Arlene and Charlie—was wheeled into the OR the following morning amid a general mood of euphoria. The story had gotten around the operating suite and everyone was happy for her, especially Dr. Wallace. Not only was Wallace one of the kindliest, most gentle people on the senior surgical staff, but it turned out that he was also an old friend and college chum of Arlene's father. She had known him all her life.

The anesthesiologist whispered some encouraging words into Arlene's ear, and she was off to a peaceful, anticipatory sleep, no doubt already looking forward to the exciting changes that would soon occur in her relationship with the man she loved so much. As soon as the breathing tube had been slid into her windpipe, the nurses put her up in stirrups and the gynecologist excised the leathery hymen in less than five minutes. I prepped the left breast with Merthiolate as Joe had taught me, and Wallace carefully excised the lump and held it for a moment in his hand before having it sent downstairs for an immediate frozen section by the pathologist. I could tell by the look that suddenly appeared in the surgeon's eyes that something was troubling him. He told Joe to close the small biopsy wound, stepped a few feet away from the table, and asked for a fresh scalpel so that he could cut into the tissue he had just removed.

"I don't like it," he murmured glumly, just loudly enough for those of us at the operating table to hear him. Those four words must have sent the same chill up everyone's backbone that they did mine, especially when they were followed a moment later by "It's gritty—it's hard." Wallace was describing a cancer.

It took fifteen minutes for the report of the frozen section to be called up to us on the intercom, and they were the longest minutes I would spend during my entire twelve weeks on the various surgical services. The pathologist's flat, emotionless voice confirmed the diagnosis of cancer, and added his observation that it "looks particularly aggressive." Joe and I wordlessly took off the biopsy drapes and prepped a wide area of the patient's chest wall and upper arm in preparation for a radical mastectomy.

It took about four hours to remove the breast and the entire contiguous mass of axillary tissue in the armpit. A skin graft was required to close the defect left in the skin by such a wide dissection. Beyond the few sentences necessary to communicate among the team, the OR was hushed. I was aware of every sigh of the anesthesia apparatus.

When the last stitch had been tied down to hold the graft in place, Wallace lay the whole specimen—that entire beautiful breast and the contents of the armpit—on a small instrument table so that he could feel the nodes contained within the axillary contents. "Palpate them, Forkner, and tell me what you think," he said, pointing to a few lymph nodes in the highest part of the axillary fat pad, farthest from the breast itself. Joe agreed that they felt hard and were almost certainly the site of cancerous spread. The little lumps thought to have been caused by a minor infection of the skin of the armpit were actually filled with malignancy. In those days, finding malignant infiltration of the highest nodes was a death sentence. What should have been a benign tumor of the breast in a vibrantly healthy young woman had revealed itself to be a destroyer of dreams, an assassin.

In a solemn procession, Wallace, Joe, and I followed behind Arlene's gurney as two orderlies wheeled it from the OR to the recovery room. It seemed only right that we should remain close to the surgeon while he waited to speak to his patient once she was fully awake, so we sat silently at a desk where interns usually write postoperative orders. Wallace never took his eyes off her.

It was barely ten minutes before Arlene woke up. When she had exchanged a few words with the nurse and had a few sips of water, Wallace laboriously lifted himself from his chair and slowly shuffled the ten paces to her side. Joe and I stayed close behind him, as though we could somehow give him strength in what he would have to do. When Arlene saw him, she smiled in the same open, sunny way she had when Joe told her of the hymenotomy that promised to change her life forever. "Isn't it wonderful that it's over," she whispered, her eyes glistening as though she were turning a glorious new page in the book of her life. Wallace hesitated for a moment before speaking, and then he said, "Arlene, there's something we have to talk about."

Commentary to
The Family Physician's Tale

The Family Physician's Tale recounts events that occurred more than half a century ago. At that time, the spread of breast cancer to the highest lymph nodes of the axilla, especially in a young woman, was a virtual death sentence. I add "virtual" because this form of malignancy is a disease whose course has always been known to have an element of individual idiosyncrasy. An occasional woman with a dire prognosis lives for decades without evidence of worsening, while the opposite is sometimes true when the odds for cure should be high.

Every tumor of every organ bears its own unknowable biological characteristics that influence the course of growth and the results of treatment, but nowhere is this more true than in malignancies of the breast. It is precisely such factors that make predictions so difficult and long-term outlook so uncertain. Nevertheless, given a large group of young women whose extent of disease was similar to that described in the Tale just told, it is certain that almost all of them, in 1955, would have been dead within three years. And so it proved to be for Arlene Williams. Within six months of operation, she developed evidence of metastasis to the liver and several ribs. She was dead a year later. No treatment known at that time could have saved her.

Things are different now. A woman with disease the extent of Arlene's would today be subjected to a far less drastic operation on her breast, sampling of the axillary nodes instead of wide excision, and courses of highly developed chemotherapy, radiation, and hormones that stand a reasonable chance of slowing or even arresting her disease for a long period of time, sometimes indefinitely. Her debility in the postoperative months would have been a great deal less than Arlene suffered with the healing radical mastectomy. After the initial courses of therapy, her quality of life would be remarkably better than Arlene's was during the majority of those final eighteen months. Moreover, and very likely of greatest importance, an Arlene of the first decade of the twenty-first century would have certainly undergone a mammogram when she first discovered the lump in her breast, or even before. Though the notion of visualizing the breast with small doses of X-ray delivered with a standard machine was first suggested in 1920, it was very infrequently used, both because of its unreliability and the general attitude of many, if not most, women that a diagnosis of breast cancer carried with it a shame and stigma difficult to bear or discuss. Even more than almost any other cancer at that time, it was rarely spoken of or admitted to. Not until the 1960s did specialized X-ray machines dedicated solely to mammography make their appearance. Radiographic diagnosis became rapidly more accurate, radiologists began to subspecialize in mammography, and X-ray criteria for biopsy and early diagnosis were developed and increasingly refined.

Another change took place soon thereafter, and it may have been of even more consequence than mammography at the time. In 1974, only a few months after her husband's inauguration as President of the United States, Betty Ford publicly announced her recent diagnosis of breast cancer and treatment with mastectomy. With her as an example, Happy Rockefeller, the wife of the Vice-President Designate, decided one day soon thereafter to examine her own breasts. She discovered a small lump that proved to be malignant, and underwent mastectomy at the Memorial Sloan-Kettering Hospital in New York. Like Mrs. Ford, she chose to tell her story to the public, in the hope that other women might be encouraged to become proactive in a situation so commonly feared and subject to secrecy and even social ignominy. The immediate—and it was indeed immediate—result of the public courage and responsibility demonstrated by these two insightful and far-seeing women encouraged many thousands if not hundreds of thousands of women to examine their own breasts, seek medical advice, and undergo mammography. A disease mired in shame suddenly became the subject of a crusade, and many lives were saved.

Even women like Arlene Williams, who was "not one to go to doctors," now began in large numbers to seek examination, with the result that many new cancers were found when still at an early and often curable stage. I so well remember remarking in the late 1970s that nothing less than a Nobel Prize in Medicine was deserved by these two courageous and civic-minded women for all they had done to remove the stigma of a frightening disease, and for serving as human catalysts for what must certainly have been a considerable number of cures. I have no doubt that a woman like Arlene would have been far less reluctant to seek medical advice about a breast lump after the mid-1970s than she was in the late 1950s. Whether she might have been cured is impossible to know, but her chances would certainly have been vastly improved with an early diagnosis.

More recently, magnetic resonance imaging scans have been added to the list of diagnostic recommendations, because they have been found to identify cancers that standard mammography and the use of ultrasound sometimes miss. The American Cancer Society now recommends that women who, for any of a variety of reasons (such as known breast cancer gene mutations or a strong family history of breast cancer), are thought to be at high risk undergo a yearly MRI in addition to the mammogram. MRI scans are especially useful in women whose breast tissue is particularly dense, containing a high proportion of glandular and connective tissue and a low amount of fat.

Shortly before I began recording The Family Physician's Tale, I received a greeting card inscribed with a message from a patient whose story is a case in point. Marie Consiglio was referred to me in 1986 by a physician in a town fifty miles from Canterbury. The doctor had been so shocked by the advanced state of her breast cancer that he could only hope that someone at a university hospital might provide some comfort and local wound hygiene to a situation worse than any he had ever encountered.

The best way to describe Marie Consiglio would be a rugged individualist who most emphatically went her own way in all things, and had never had much regard for the medical profession. I always suspected that her combination of personal toughness and an aggressively keen intelligence hid a deeply submerged fear of serious disease, but I have no way of proving that; our many conversations over the subsequent years revealed not a clue to support my thesis—no clue, that is, except the presence before me of a savvy woman who did not seek medical attention for her cancer until it was so advanced that it had ulcerated through the skin and putrefied a significant portion of the tissue of her right breast. Had Marie been married, there is no doubt that her husband would have long since demanded that she see a doctor. But in this as in all other matters, this attractive, witty—and here I must use the word "desirable"—woman had made her own choice, and it was to remain single despite what I assume must have been the pursuit of more than a few suitors.

To put it in most direct terms: Marie Consiglio's breast was a mess. Surgery could not be curative; it would require the removal of a great deal of tissue right down to the rib cage merely to achieve a satisfactory degree of healing. And even if the healing somehow took place without complex postoperative infection, the best that could be hoped for was cosmetic: The mess would be removed, but the usual biology of breast cancer meant that undiscoverable tumor (one could only hope that it was more microscopic than bulky) must certainly remain elsewhere in her body.

What to do? I consulted with colleagues in radiotherapy and oncology, and together we devised a plan of action that we thought might stand some chance of providing a few years of symptom-free life until Marie's inevitable death. This involved carefully designed courses of chemotherapy and radiation before surgery was even considered. This part of the protocol took months to administer but was effective in rendering the breast operable. When all the preoperative therapies had been completed, I did a wide mastectomy, the wound healed without complication, and the oncologist took over again. An optimist by nature, he was by now becoming encouraged to think in terms of long-term survival, and he accordingly released into his patient's bloodstream whatever therapeutic poisons he felt were required to accomplish his objective.

I stopped doing Marie's follow-up examinations five years later, in 1992 when I began my writing career, but she has been closely observed by physicians in her home city. She and I exchange letters from time to time and occasionally see each other briefly, so I have been able to keep close track of her condition—which remains remarkably healthy.

The words inscribed on Marie's greeting card tell the story of a series of treatments for what was certainly, at the time of Arlene Williams's presentation, a hopeless situation. Her card begins with the words "Hello, dear old buddy—Thought it appropriate on the 20th anniversary of my surgery to drop a note of thanks. Life is great . . . ." Marie is without evidence of cancer. The situation for women with advanced disease has become even better since she first appeared in my office in 1986, and I suspect it will become better still in the next few decades, as new chemotherapeutic and perhaps immunological treatments are developed.

When the Family Physician had completed the narration of his Tale, I asked him if he had any information about whether the hymenotomy had made a difference in the months following operation. Had it enabled two such deeply committed people to achieve at least some small bit of unanticipated happiness as they faced the inevitability that loomed before them? His reply was what I expected: He did not know.

CR

The Dermatologist's Tale

DERMATOLOGISTS ARE NOT NOTED for the excitement aroused by their case reports. And I suppose that not many readers of my Tale will disagree, once they reach its very unexciting climax. But that's the entire point of writing about our specialty: to take what would seem a minor problem for the vast majority of people not afflicted by it, and point out how solving it for one individual changes that person's life.

I came to Canterbury to do research and teach, but I spend about half of my time seeing patients. Most of them are referred from elsewhere, for diagnosis and treatment of those "minor problems" that plague patient and doctor alike. One of them was the forty-two-year-old woman about whom I am writing here. Joan Carson had no medical problems except the one that I call her "needle in a haystack," which was a mysterious rash on her upper eyelids. She had first noticed redness and swelling of the lids about three months earlier, which she assumed was caused by her makeup, although she had not recently changed it. She visited a dermatologist, who began treatment in the standard fashion with a series of cortisone products and antihistamines. In a relatively short time, the condition so worsened that Mrs. Carson could no longer go to her job as an executive secretary because, as her boss explained to her, "the rash makes the whole office look sick, and wearing dark glasses only makes our operation a little suspect to newcomers."

Using steroids by mouth and then intramuscularly did not change the situation at all. Having exhausted what she thought were all the resources of allopathic, or orthodox, medicine, Mrs. Carson was on the verge of seeking help from a nonlicensed practitioner when her dermatologist suggested that she try a consultation at Canterbury, which is the route by which many of my patients come to me and to my colleagues in the department: Few people visit a university dermatologist directly as a first choice, there being so many able ones in most cities.

On her initial visit, Mrs. Carson tearfully expressed grave doubts that I could help her. I've long been inured to such occasionally correct comments and proceed anyway, because patience and a willingness to try tedious diagnostic methods and unusual therapies are the hallmark of us academic types, and are often our main means of succor when equally able specialists have failed.

Though I suspected contact dermatitis, there were no obvious culprits, and all but three patch tests were negative. Two of them tested over-the-counter antibiotics that she had used for self-treatment, each of which had actually worsened her condition. The third was for a chemical called dimethylaminoproylamine, or DMAPA, an ingredient whose name was completely unfamiliar to me—but not for long. A few minutes of online research revealed that DMAPA was a chemical produced by the breakdown of cocamidopropyl betaine (CPB), a surfactant widely used in shampoos and liquid soaps. A few calls to the manufacturer of Mrs. Carson's favorite shampoo and conditioner did indeed show that it contained CPB, and accordingly was the cause of her rare form of dermatitis. What may be most remarkable is that she had been using the same hair-care product for years, with no difficulty. But since switching to an equally effective alternative, she has never had another problem. DMAPA caused by the chemical reaction of CPB was like an old friend who had deserted her—her needle in a haystack within another haystack.

As promised, it's a (seemingly) simple story with a (seemingly) simple solution, and it doesn't even require a Commentary by the Narrator.

૭ం

The Gastroenterologist's Tale

MONG THE MANY REWARDS of being a gastroenterologist is the wide age range of patients who come to me for consultation and treatment. Of course, some of my colleagues do specialize in small children, and I have chosen a cutoff age of ten, but beyond this, I might call myself a family physician of diseases of the stomach, intestines, and their associated organs, including the liver and gallbladder.

I practice at a hospital located in an area of a large city known for its population of Holocaust survivors, and this sometimes takes a kind of thoughtfulness and discretion that I have tried to learn over these many years. Every once in a while a situation arises that is unique to this group, and I try not only to ameliorate it but also to use it as a lesson in the humanity required of us as healers of people who may long ago have lost faith in the form of authority represented by physicians.

The first of the cases I have chosen to describe falls into this category while the second is of quite a different sort, though they both illustrate a point so often made by the Narrator, namely that medicine is an uncertain art. No matter how carefully we analyze the subgroups we study so assiduously in our research and literature, we always get back to the maxim first elucidated by Hippocrates and even today followed by experienced physicians: that each individual brings his or her own packet of riddles that must be solved. When people have undergone traumas unknown to the vast majority of us—as has my first patient—the packet is likely to be larger and its contents more varied.

Aaron Schultheis was an elderly man who had been admitted to the hospital several days earlier for the evaluation of severe osteoarthritis of the hips and knees. As the students on bedside rounds went through the usual litany of causes for such a major disability—genetics, trauma, overuse—a girl in the group asked him about Auschwitz. Having met the patient the day before, she knew that he was a survivor of six years at that notorious camp and asked that he tell about the conditions he had suffered there. Though he had seemed stoic at first, his manner changed completely as he described the bitter cold, the lack of proper clothes in the harsh winters, and the generally dreadful conditions he had had to endure. And then he asked the obvious question: "Could any of this have caused the breakdown in my joints?" Before the attending physician, Joe Curtis, could begin to answer, the old man broke down in wracking sobs: "My whole family was killed! I left nineteen of them there, and I'm the only one left." It was as though he had been transported to a different place, a different atmosphere, and a completely different time in his life. "Where can I go? What can I do? Where will they send me next?"

Joe held the old man's hands in his own, but the gesture somehow seemed insufficient. Within moments, he had leaned forward and was rocking the patient's entire body in his arms. "You're here with us, Mr. Schultheis. This is your home now; no one can ever send you away again. You're in America, and it is safe." The old man held tight to Joe for a minute or two, as if to convince himself that this was no fantasy he was hearing. And then he slowly let go, looked directly at the doctor—thirty years his junior—and came back to this moment and this place, and to Joe.

This most memorable patient Joe had ever seen taught *me* yet another lesson, one similar to the Narrator's aphorism and to the one I learned from the young woman whose story I will relate a bit further on. It has to do with the individuality of people and the necessity to cast the rules aside when they seem to make little sense for the person sitting before you at a given moment in his or her life and yours.

Laboratory testing a few days later showed a trace of blood in Mr. Schultheis's stool, repeatedly on three occasions. The usual protocol requires at least a sigmoidoscopy to determine the presence of a polyp or worse, so I was asked to see him for that purpose. In view of his frailty, I used a minimal clean-out prep and discovered a four-centimeter polyp about eighteen centimeters from the opening of his anus. Microscopic evaluation of the biopsy revealed a small focus of malignancy. The next step was to recommend an operation, because the base of the polyp was too broad to remove it through my scope. We were still in the days before such procedures could be done laparoscopically, so I asked one of my surgical colleagues to do a short excision of the involved area. We both agreed that this was an appropriate measure, so the procedure was scheduled for a few days hence. Though his cardiac workup had seemed satisfactory, even the induction of anesthesia proved to be too much for our patient, who had a cardiac arrest from which he could not be resuscitated.

My geriatrician colleagues came down hard on me, and they were justified to do so. They showed me well-documented evidence in their literature indicating that the life expectancy of a frail eighty-five-year-old man was approximately three years, far less than I could justify by my ill-considered decision to recommend operation for a man with a minimally invasive polyp that would almost certainly not have taken his life within that time. It was a case of bad judgment, and I have no excuse for it. To compound the injury, I had not only failed to consult with them prior to recommending surgery, but had downplayed its dangers when speaking to Mr. Schultheis.

Not really to balance my poor decision-making in the case of Mr. Schultheis, I do have another sort of Tale to relate, which in its own way tells the opposite story. It is of a situation in which I defied the standards of the time (about fifteen years ago) and turned out to be right. I was consulted by a twenty-eight-year-old woman who was concerned because her father had just been diagnosed with colon cancer at age fifty-five. She had been reading a great deal about the necessity of evaluating close family members under such circumstances and wanted to be colonoscoped. Both at that time and today, colonoscopy at such a young age, regardless of family history, was not being advocated, but for reasons of which I'm still not certain I decided to go ahead with the procedure. To my amazement the woman proved to have a small polyp in her transverse colon, with an early malignancy. I took out the polyp and have followed her since that time, with no evidence of recurrence.

The Obstetrician-Gynecologist's Tale

THIS IS THE SECOND Tale involving the specialty of Obstetrics and Gynecology in this book, but it's the only one written by a real obstetrician, so I claim some priority. This memorable situation occurred in my early days of clinical work in the 1980s when I was in a group that included four obstetricians—all but one a woman—and a variety of specialists from other fields. We were all participants in a community health plan that eventually had to close down for lack of support from the very groups who had asked that it be established in their small city.

Jean Tucker was an army wife, and this was her first pregnancy. Because her husband was frequently transferred, she had
received care at several bases, and we were having some difficulty
obtaining her old records. The only thing we knew was due to
her having told us that she was "born with something wrong with
my female organs," but our exams and ultrasounds didn't show
anything of consequence. Because Jean's care was spread among
the four of us, no one really took charge to aggressively pursue
the records, especially since everything seemed so normal.

One of the striking personality characteristics I admired in
Jean was her sense of equanimity. I've had few patients in my
practice who approached a first delivery with the calm she so
obviously possessed. Being a bit of a nervous Nelly myself, and
perhaps knowing too much, I had been quite the opposite as my
own first child's birth approached, so I was even more impressed
with Jean than I might otherwise have been. Accordingly, you
can imagine my surprise when, on the actual day of delivery, she
arrived on the labor floor emotionally out of control and unable
to bear the pain. What was even more surprising was that her cervix was still closed and thick—she was not at all dilated. I gave her
a small dose of morphine, but it had little effect on her response
to what I would have expected to be a relatively minor amount
of significant discomfort. In fact, when she awoke from a brief
nap, she was agitated and inconsolable with misery despite an
unchanged cervix. Remarkably, she would allow me to examine
her only when she was on all fours, a truly unusual situation.

To my absolute amazement, I found a fully dilated cervix
when I examined her in this position. It took a slow, careful

evaluation before I realized what I was dealing with: Jean had a double vagina from the cervix to the hymeneal ring, the two parts separated by a wall or septum. The cervix through which she had conceived was wide open, and the baby's head was close to crowning.

Unfortunately, the septum was so thick and filled with blood vessels that I was unable to stretch it sufficiently to deliver the baby. A decision had to be made, and it had to be made quickly. One of the anesthesiologists gave Jean an epidural to keep her from the urge to push, and we took her down to the operating room. Once there, I began cutting away enough of the septum to allow the vagina to dilate sufficiently for a safe delivery. This was a tricky maneuver, because the baby, head full of wet hair and covered with the usual glop, was trying to come down the vagina even as I was providing room for it, making for a bit of competition between nature and surgery. But all worked out well, a healthy baby was delivered, and the residual pieces of septum later scarred into small shrunken bits. The happy outcome was that I delivered two more of Jean's children in the next five years, without a bit of problem.

The Ophthalmologist's Tale

F YOU'RE EXPECTING A Tale about eyeballs or retinitis pigmentosa, you're sure to be disappointed. Actually, I might just as well have entitled this little story The Obstetrician's Tale, because it is the adventure of my unintended foray into that specialty, during the time I was fulfilling my military obligation in the mid-1950s. The older doctors who read this piece will recall a twisted bit of logic (in all fairness, some thought it was a great idea) called the Berry Plan.

The basic principles of the plan devised by General Frank Berry—who was appointed secretary of Defense and director of the Selective Service System (pronounced "draft") in 1954—

were relatively straightforward. Some way had to be found that would provide for the huge cold-war medical needs of the U.S. military while interfering as little as possible with the specialty training of those physicians who were a part of it. The obvious solution for obtaining the manpower was to threaten doctors with being drafted at the end of their internship unless they enlisted; the solution for the bit of kindness was to allow the enlistees to choose the two-year period in which they elected to serve. Since the interns declining to enlist faced almost certain draft, the Berry Plan, though really a Hobson's choice, was a popular one.

The system interlocked very well with the system of specialty training of that time. Having graduated from medical school and completed an internship, most doctors enrolled in a residency training program, some as short as the two to three years required for pediatrics and others as long as the perhaps six or seven for neurosurgery in those long-ago days. Of course, today's programs are a lot longer, because they encompass a wider knowledge base and usually require at least one year spent in the research lab. But to be posted in some interesting European or Asian country for two years at the rank of captain was not considered a great hardship, especially because provision was made for the expenses of wife and children. One could live a very comfortable life in a place like England or Germany, buy all necessary provisions at the cheap prices available on the base, and have plenty of time to travel. If lucky enough, a young doctor might even find himself posted to a hospital where he could learn a great deal about the specialty he would later study.

I had married just after college graduation, and the end of my internship found Marilyn and me with three children under the age of four. At $25 a month, my fifty-two weeks of working every other night had left me not only destitute, but in debt to Marilyn's father for several thousand dollars we had had to borrow, not to mention a significant pile-up of tuition expense. The Berry Plan may have seemed a form of coercion to some of my bachelor colleagues, but Marilyn and I saw it as a bonanza. At two years of a captain's salary, I could wipe out my debts and have a bit of a nest egg for my three-year residency in eye surgery. And the odds were good that I'd be stationed in a fascinating place (I was hoping for Denmark) and we could live like Lord and Lady Rosenzweig, instead of two impoverished debtors from the Bronx owing money to a diabetic tie salesman.

We leaped at the opportunity. I signed the papers as soon as they were processed and sent to me during the second month of my internship, in August 1955. Because neither of us had ever been south of Hackensack, New Jersey, the words "Gunter Air Force Base" emblazoned on my post–basic training orders were very exciting to read. Gunter was situated in a town called Montgomery, Alabama, and that had a nice ring to it as well. A peacefully quiet southern city for three weeks of orientation and then we'd be on a plane across the Atlantic to our final posting. During those three weeks, I'd be given my captain's bars, learn how to be an officer, and then be handed my treasured European assignment.

By the time we arrived there, Montgomery was not, of course, a peacefully quiet southern city. A thirty-nine-year-old seamstress named Rosa Parks had changed all of that during the previous December. The bus boycott was in full swing, and it would not end until after the Supreme Court made its historic decision in November. It was a very exciting time to be in a place I'd never heard of until only the year before.

Neither Marilyn nor I was a stranger to racial bigotry. There was plenty of it in the North, though our experience of it had taken a significantly different form than what we witnessed on the streets and in the shops and public places of Montgomery, where the boycott brought out facets of people's characters that must have been shocking even to themselves. Gunter itself was split among those who supported the strikers, those who opposed them, and the small group that took no interest whatsoever. Though no one in uniform dared take part in the demonstrations, a few of our number made their feelings clear by their behavior on the base. I found myself far more involved than my fantasies of Denmark might have predicted.

The expectation of being at Gunter for the usual short period exploded in my face one day during the early part of the third week. I was thumbing through one of the army medical manuals when a sergeant called out to tell me that I was wanted immediately by Colonel Ransom, the officer in charge of my unit. Though still a fledgling in the Air Force, several truths had already become clear to me. One was the meaning of that word "immediately," which was better interpreted as "as soon as you get a free moment." Another was that a summons to the boss's office will almost never result in anything good. And the third applied to me personally: I was the only Jew—and with a Bronx accent untouched by four years at Canterbury and an internship at the Boston City Hospital, no less—in the unit, and the colonel was a first-class anti-Semite. The only group he hated more than Jews were blacks, and he never lost the opportunity to say so. He never overtly said a word against Jews, but he didn't have to: I had long since learned the signs and symptoms, and he had all of them.

But he responded differently to Negroes—which is the word we customarily used in those days. The bus boycott had turned his constant low flame of loathing and contempt into a roaring bonfire that he fed with every bit of combustible fury in his southern soul. It was as though Harry Ransom had been trained in some academy of hate in his hometown of Lakeside, Mississippi, and he wanted everyone to know it. He was unrestrained not only in his words, but in his actions. Though he could not, as a uniformed officer in the United States Air Force, do anything about the bus boycott, he could take out his wrath on the few black non-coms in our unit—and he did. Yet even this did not satisfy him. All of these young men were from the South, and no indignity was either new to them or unexpected, so his vituperations were for naught. He must have felt as if his soul were being bathed in a constant sulfurous liquid of frustration: His Negroes didn't care, and he could do nothing overt about his one Jew. But the summons to his office made me wonder whether he had figured out some way to relieve himself of at least some small bit of his exploding wrath. Turned out that my Jew-boy intuition was on precisely the right wavelength.

"Take a seat, Captain, take a seat," Ransom said as soon as I had snapped my newly learned salute. He spoke in tones so thickly southern that he might as well have been a caricature. The first time I'd heard him, addressing our unit on arrival, I was sure he was playing a joke on us, as if to say, "Now boys, here's how a *real* Reb talks!" But he did indeed talk in this accent. Had he spoken that way in a college play, he'd have lost the role for overacting, but for Colonel Hartigan Thibodeaux Ransom, this was the real thing.

"I have some news you're going to like," he began, which that Jew-boy intuition told me was some news I wouldn't like. "You, you lucky fellow, you get to stay here at Gunter for your whole two years. I've decided you're too valuable to waste out at Landstuhl in Germany or one of those other jobs anybody can do. As you know, Gunter is the Air Force Medical School, and I need you to stay here and be an instructor in Public Health and Preventive Medicine."

I sputtered a few "buts," which helped me not at all, because Ransom had the perfect response, accompanied by the smug smile of a victory won. "We've never had an officer here from Canterbury, and you do know that's the best Public Health department in the country, so you're my man."

And that's how I came to be scheduled for two hopeless years in Montgomery, Alabama. The only good thing about it was that I was able to find myself a job moonlighting several nights a week in the emergency room of a small local hospital, where the pay was good and not much work needed to be done. Still, I was bored beyond description.

One night toward the end of my first year, a girl of about fifteen came in accompanied by her mother. Though she checked in under the name of Laura Taylor, I recognized the mother immediately as Harry Ransom's wife, Hester. I had been told that Ransom's daughter, Laura, was away at boarding school, so I'd never seen her before. And since both she and her mother knew who I was, the whole situation was fraught with embarrassment for everyone. This place was, of course, not the excellent teaching hospital at Gunter, but a little suburban facility with few sophisticated specialists on call.

The girl was writhing with severe abdominal pain, and her belly was markedly distended. Though it's unusual for people with peritonitis to move around very much, I wondered whether she might have ruptured her appendix. But when I touched that hard, bloated protuberance, I felt the unmistakable rolling sensation of uterine contractions. I thought the outraged Mrs. Ransom would hit me with her pocketbook when I asked whether Laura might be pregnant, but there was no alternative to the question. Laura herself cried softly and turned her head from side to side signifying the utter impossibility of such a thing.

I insisted on calling the obstetrician—and did—but Mrs. Ransom indignantly told me that she was taking Laura to Gunter, where she would not be insulted by such impertinence. The whole situation had by now become ridiculous, because Gunter was where she should have gone in the first place. I suspected that their real destination was to be Tuskegee, about twelve miles away. It would have taken a lot of swallowed pride to do such a thing, but there seemed no alternative. They headed for the door in spite of my protestations, with Laura still on the gurney.

As they approached the outer exit, I heard a shout from one of the nurses: "Something's coming out!" I ran toward them, pulling the sheet off the girl to find that between her thighs a small brown foot was protruding. The nurse and I prepared to deliver the rest of the child, which was lying in what obstetricians call the double footling position. Fortunately, I had had experience with a case like this when I was a medical student on the obstetric service at Canterbury, so I knew just what to do. I was able to extract the baby rather easily, because I remembered the maneuver and the baby was very small. I pulled out the other foot, straddled the baby on my arm, and inserted my finger in the lower jaw so the head did not become caught on the pelvic rim of this petite mother. It was at this point that the obstetrician arrived and had the sad responsibility of telling Mrs. Ransom that the baby was a stillborn.

I never said a word to anyone except Marilyn about that night. But a day later, I was called into the colonel's office and told that my orders were to be changed. I was to be assigned to Landstuhl, the great Air Force base in Germany, where I was to complete my period of service. As I stepped into the corridor, Ransom said a few more words: "And I'm sure you know what I expect of you, Rosenzweig." I nodded and left.

❧

Commentary to
The Ophthalmologist's Tale

Stan Rosenzweig hardly needed those parting words from the colonel. Of course, he could have told the story all over Gunter, in a kind of sweet revenge on behalf of every Negro, Jew, and minority of any kind who had ever been the subject of Ransom's abuse or even of his barely hidden contempt. But Stan was not that kind of man. In fact, what he felt for his commanding officer—and for the man's family, too—was pity of a sort. He never saw any of them again, but it was years before he was able to stop thinking about them every single day.

What must it have been like for Ransom to know that his cuddled, coddled, and much-loved daughter was pregnant? I'll guess that he was never told the race of the child's father, nor could he have imagined that the young man could possibly be black. Or perhaps I'm wrong. Perhaps the pregnancy was the result of a real teenage love affair, and Ransom knew precisely who the child's father was. And while I'm perhapsing, perhaps he was filled with remorse that his grandson was stillborn. I run a scenario through my mind—doubtless completely unrealistic—that Ransom was transformed by this event; that he spoke to the boy with kindness and even sympathy; that he not only allowed the romance to continue but actually encouraged it; that Laura's children of the eventual marriage were raised in a loving home, and that they grew up to become fighters for civil rights, using their grandfather's reformation as an example of what might happen even in the most bigoted of hearts. What I have been describing would have been an impossibility in the South of the 1950s. Even today, the idea of such a thing seems wildly fanciful. A novel based on such a premise would be rejected by every publisher.

An irony of this Tale is that Stan feels no particular pride in keeping Ransom's secret. It's what he believes any man of integrity would have done. But to properly deliver a double footling—a type of breech in which the feet present first—when one has had no more training than six weeks as a medical student on obstetrics, that's a story he has often told.

CR

The Cardiologist's Tale

I'VE ALWAYS BEEN INTERESTED in the early history of the printed book, especially the volumes that appeared in the decades soon after the invention of moveable type by Johannes Gutenberg around the middle of the fifteenth century. At least two or three times a year, I walk over to Canterbury's rare book library and stand—reverentially, you might say—for a few minutes before the large and specially designed case where the curators have set up a permanent exhibit of the university's copy of one of the few Gutenberg Bibles still in existence. Until only months before his death in 2000, Joe Dennet had always been there to greet me. Even as his health was rapidly failing during the last few years of his life, he would sometimes have a taxi bring him to his office in the library, always finding some bit of work to do, which, he never failed to assure me, "might not be thought of by someone else." And, because I usually let him know when I was planning a visit, he'd have an assistant prepare one or two incunabula for me to look at, those books printed between the time of Gutenberg's invention and 1500, even if he could not be there himself to show it to me.

I loved my visits with Joe, whether in the library or during the time we spent together in my outpatient office, where I tried desperately during his last four years of life to ameliorate his ever-worsening congestive heart failure. He had first become my patient in 1982 when, at the age of fifty-seven, he was brought into the emergency room with a major heart attack, soon to be followed by a series of complications requiring that a balloon pump be inserted in his aorta for maintenance of the blood supply to his cardiac circulation. Though he was temporarily stabilized by that procedure, it proved insufficient, and one afternoon he had to be rushed to the operating room for an urgent coronary artery bypass graft of three vessels.

Remarkably, Joe did well for about fifteen years, working every day and not needing to relinquish his duties as director of the rare book library until the mandatory retirement age of seventy. About a year after that, he had another myocardial infarction while on vacation in Colorado. When he returned to Canterbury after a prolonged stay at a hospital in Denver, it was obvious that he was in mild-to-moderate congestive heart failure, which continued to worsen over the next four years of his life in spite of every measure I and my colleagues took to control it. To complicate matters, he developed a disturbance of cardiac rhythm requiring the implantation of a defibrillator, without which his heart could not maintain an effective beat on its own.

Joe had led a fascinating life. Not only had he negotiated major bequests of money, manuscripts, and books to the school, but the stories of his acquisition of many of the library's treasures had become the stuff of legend among knowledgeable people. He had matched wits not only with a few of the most colorful dealers of his time in countries on several continents, but personally with the likes of the Vanderbilts and Whitneys, as well as a host of far less savory characters who had in one or another way come into possession of some of the most rare and valuable literary gems in existence. Many were the stories he told me of having to track down the provenance of a book or manuscript before being sure that it had been acquired honestly by the often shady, secretive, and equally often flamboyant character or characters from whom he needed to purchase it.

Even had Joe not kept scrupulous official records of each transaction, his prodigious memory was a file of fascination, including certain intimate impressions of various sorts of book people—impressions of the sort that never find their way into the written records of a university's collections. He was a skilled negotiator, a shrewd bargainer, and, when absolutely necessary, even a bit of a con artist. But, as he assured me on more than one occasion, "I always stayed on the right side of the law and what is considered ethics in our strange trade, though sometimes by just a bit." Joe had good reason to be proud of his accomplishments: The university had been immeasurably enriched by his career, and he left its collections—only average when he came to them in his late twenties—among the greatest in the world. But every once in a while, especially as his condition worsened, he would confide regret that with his passing, virtually all the lore in his well-ordered store of personal mental recollections would go with him to the grave.

Joe's heart failure finally reached the point where he had to stop even those occasional expeditions to the small office maintained for him in the library. Our clinical visits became more frequent, near the end going from once a month to weekly. This was not because I had anything new to offer, but I hoped that seeing him so often might strengthen his tattered spirits, even if a little. And I had another motivation, which was hardly unselfish: I wanted to see this one-of-a-kind man—who had by then long been as much a friend as a patient—more often when the final days of his life began to approach. As his, and my, hopes dwindled, I sought a stratagem to ease his lengthy period of emotional anguish in any way I could.

And then one day I hit on it. At the end of one of Joe's weekly visits, I handed him a new prescription blank. He expressed surprise at having been given it, because, except for refills, some long time had passed since I had any new medications or changes in therapy to offer. But his eyes brightened as he looked down at the small bit of paper with "Rx" inscribed on its upper left-hand corner. The prescription I had given Joe consisted of four words:

"One set of memoirs." As his eyes lingered on it for a moment, his face lit up with the first smile I had seen in many months, and even his labored breathing seemed to become easier for a minute or more. He left the office with a cheery, "I've told you a few of these stories, but even you will be surprised at what's in this book, I promise you."

Within days, Joe had begun dictating to his daughter-in-law for hours at a time each day, and she was so pleased at the change in him that she was willing to devote as much time to the work as his cardiac insufficiency and breathing difficulties allowed. The project moved more quickly than I could have imagined; each time he came to see me, he had not only progress to report but a sense of purpose I had not seen in him since I first told him that we had run out of therapeutic options. Though nothing in his clinical condition or prognosis had improved, he seemed a different man as the work proceeded. As much as I rejoiced in his new attitude, I dreaded the day when the pages would be completed. In fact, I would occasionally hint that he ought to move more slowly, but Joe was taking no chances on leaving so much as half a chapter undone.

A little more than three months after he had begun his assignment, Joe's wife brought him in for one of his regular weekly appointments. Though he could not complete a spoken sentence without stopping several times for breath, he looked up at me from his wheelchair with an expression of what I can only call triumph. Tucked under his arm was the first photocopy of the manuscript of his completed memoirs. He had dedicated it to me. Centered on page one was a copy of the prescription.

The memoir was complete, and Joe Dennet was ready to die. But there was to be one more office visit. Neither Joe nor I wanted his death to be the result of congestive heart failure, which is like slow drowning as the lungs fill with fluid. Reluctant as I was to say the words, I offered to contact the electrophysiology laboratory to have his defibrillator turned off. Joe knew that only this mechanical device stood between him and an irregularity of cardiac rhythm that would take his life within a very few minutes, but without suffering. He accepted, and the laboratory appointment was made for three days later.

Joe Dennet died suddenly and painlessly at home, two hours before the scheduled appointment to turn off his defibrillator.

∞

Commentary to *The Cardiologist's Tale*

To some, the climax of The Cardiologist's Tale would represent a problem in medical ethics. In their view, to turn off a defibrillator is a form of active euthanasia—similar to physician-assisted suicide—in which an act is committed with the deliberate intent of ending a life. To others, it would fall into the category of a more passive deed: A man is being kept alive, though barely, by artificial means; to discontinue those means is merely to let nature take its course. But how far back in Joe Dennet's course would the latter group go? Would they have denied him the balloon pump—certainly an artificial device—that enabled him to live fifteen rewarding years? Or the coronary bypass grafts?

No one who has followed the vigorous bioethical discussions of the past four decades would agree to such decisions. Good medical and ethical care demand that every effort be expended to save a still-hopeful life, and continued unless the patient himself has expressed, in writing, his wish that further therapy be stopped should it result in a form of suffering he would not choose to endure.

Society and government have tried to solve these and similar problems with legislation that provides maximum protection and autonomy to each person who can visualize a moment when such a decision must be made. The Patient Self-Determination Act of 1990 represents the ultimate in such autonomy, allowing the spelling out of conditions— being placed on a permanent respirator or feeding tube, for example, or unequivocal evidence of an irreversible vegetative state—under which all treatment must end. By the provisions of this act, anyone while still well may designate what is called a Health Care Proxy to make such a determination should he or she become too disabled to do it, or appoint someone with a Durable Power of Attorney under similar circumstances.

I have witnessed situations in which an attorney or other proxy cannot bring himself to stop futile treatment even though the conditions are carefully spelled out in advance directives, not only empowering but by force of law ordering him to do it; I have witnessed situations in which a son or daughter long estranged from a dying parent and the entire family refuses to let the order go through, for whatever personal reason he or she may have; I have seen advance directives frustrated by a legal disagreement over an estate. In short, on more than a few occasions, I have been witness to situations in which the suffering of a dying man or woman is worsened, even though the person's wishes are spelled out in clear legal language.

It is for such reasons that the mere filling out of an advance directives form is not enough. Insofar as possible, every involved family member must be part of a conversation in which all conditions are made clear under which the attestor would no longer wish to continue living. And even that may not be enough when there remain differences between surviving family members.

Joe Dennet had no advance directives. That was a choice he made deliberately, fully aware that it might result in some form of legal hassle at the end of his life. But he had something far better—a devoted and very close-knit family, each member of which knew his precise wishes as he came closer to death. And he had Louis Kronberg, the cardiologist who told me this Tale. Though some appear to ignore or be unaware of it, all physicians have a pastoral role in the care of each patient entrusted to them. They should be guides, wise counselors, and medical advocates. Above all, they need to understand their patients as well as possible under the conditions in which the relationship has been formed. In previous eras, such a relationship often existed between family physicians and those for whom they cared—their flock, as it were. In today's highly specialized biomedicine, such a thing is much more unusual. But during fifteen years of attentive care, a friendship based on mutual interests, and the understanding that grows out of a constant and prolonged battle against disease, a pastoral quality had endured and grown between these two men. When they and Joe's wife sat down to talk about final options, advance directives were unnecessary and even superfluous. Joe was to avoid the anguish of death from congestive heart failure; Lou knew exactly how to accomplish their mutual objective. Though Lou was spared the necessity of implementing the plan on which they both agreed, no bioethics committee and no court would have had reason to criticize the act to which they had committed themselves.

The Pediatric
Cardiologist's Tale

A S A CANTERBURY GRADUATE, I, the Narrator, am sure
the pediatric cardiologist, Jim Hartenberg, would have
wanted the following Tale included in this collection,
so I'm telling it for him though he died about a decade ago, of
malignant melanoma.

For too many years, Canterbury's surgery department was in
keen competition with a great university center called Hastings,
about a hundred years older and an equal number of miles south
on the East Coast.

In virtually any other department, the schools ran neck
and neck both scientifically and clinically, though it must be

admitted that Canterbury almost always succeeded in outdoing its larger and respected neighbor in the area of heart surgery. The reasons were historical. Carl Swenson, as fearless a physician as could be found anywhere, was among the first to attempt all the new cardiac operations as they came to light in the 1940s and '50s, but Joe Cannon, the chief at Hastings, had little interest in operating on the heart. Trained as a classical lung and esophagus surgeon before World War II, he was more than a bit reluctant to dissect among the huge vessels in the upper chest. Not only that, but the first two times he operated on a ductus arteriosus proved so much more difficult and demanding than expected that he was unwilling to do more surgery on the heart.

Cannon was prepared to fall a few years behind in heart surgery when Swenson sent him a young man just finishing his general surgery training at Canterbury who had become interested in the dissection of blood vessels, in spite of being somewhat less than adept at other branches of surgery. Cannon accepted the young man as chief of his cardiac service, though he knew that a few years of ripening would be necessary to make a complete chest surgeon of him.

Richard Custis Krane gradually built his reputation on the new operations that Cannon chose not to perform. His methods in the operating room were very slow and meticulous, his patients having been carefully selected as those most likely to do well. He was not technically clumsy, but neither was he outstandingly dexterous. Krane knew little about surgical aspects of the esophagus and barely more about those of the lung. But of much more importance was that he knew his limitations and just how far he was able to go, which was more than could be said about many of his colleagues. Those early days of heart surgery were a bit like the tales told of the Wild West, with great rewards for courage but early annihilation for those who persistently took on more than they could handle.

Krane's stature rose as the years passed, and he gradually became known not only for his good results, but for introducing certain innovative procedures as well. But to be his patient required exposing oneself to certain strains beyond the usual ones of undergoing a major operation. The main problem was his clinical timidity, not generally a useful characteristic in a heart surgeon. Certain of the high risks that had to be taken with the sicker patients absolutely terrified him. Also, if he was not in the precise mood to do a particular procedure on a given day, he would cancel it on the very morning of surgery. He developed such a reputation for this kind of behavior that Cannon not only tolerated it but incorporated it into his image of the man, primarily because his operative results were in general so good.

Another of Krane's idiosyncrasies was his surgical technique. He had carefully studied everything that might conceivably go wrong in every operation he did, and devised a preventive strategy designed to keep it from happening. The one-in-a-thousand opportunity for error was never encountered in Krane's OR. The consequence of this way of operating was that lots of technical maneuvers were done that a more secure or intrepid surgeon would have avoided, and it necessitated an operating time about twice as long as would otherwise have been required. But it certainly did decrease his mortality figures and enhance his results. Krane had the longest list of successful ductus arte-riosus operations in the world, and similar feats for several other procedures.

For me as an assistant resident on his service, working with Krane in the OR was tedious, and caring for his postoperative patients even worse. Though his postops almost always did well, he had such a long list of persnickety ways in which things had to be done that to be part of his team was to study and per-form ritualistic behavior for most of the working day. We did learn a great deal, but too much was about the surgeon himself, and his quirks.

For example, we all knew that Krane had numerous ways of avoiding an operation for which he believed himself not to be temperamentally ready on a given day. He had everyday methods of avoidance that usually proved useful, though they maddened his pediatric and medical colleagues: A blood test was slightly abnormal; the patient's child had a sniffle the day before; a faint four-day-old rash on the thigh of a pediatric patient had not completely faded—these kinds of things.

But when Krane became really desperate and could think of nothing more obvious, he would use the hidden-instrument method: Send the residents in various directions to retrieve a crucial bit of equipment without which the operation was impos-sible. Off they would go, ransacking every place in the surgical pavilion where a small or large piece of highly designed stainless steel might find its way, anywhere from the most obvious cabinet to the nurses' locker room. The one predictable factor in each such episode was that the instrument would never be found, even though Krane himself combed his own office from top to bottom. The patient would have to be discharged, weeks would go by, and then the thing would reveal its location as though by some miracle. A hurried call would then be made to the anxious patient, who would scurry back in and have the operation first thing on the following morning—unless, of course, his eight-year-old had had a sniffle within the past week.

But one day the stratagem did not work, and thereon hangs the Tale. Patty Crawford was a three-year-old girl with a condition called pulmonary stenosis, which in her case meant that there was extreme narrowing of the valve separating the right side of the heart from the lungs. The result in such children is poor oxygenation, inadequate growth and development, and often a bluish tinge to the skin because of the low oxygen level in the blood; there is a limit to length of life. Krane had been following Patty as an outpatient for far too long, always waiting for what he called "the proper timing for the operation" but in fact afraid to go ahead, fearing the reported mortality rate in such patients of more than 50 percent. Perhaps it is uncharitable to say so, but there were those among the pediatric staff who wondered whether Krane would have preferred the child die without operation rather than as the result of an unsuccessful attempt at his hands.

Finally, after much badgering by Cannon, Swenson, and many of the staff, Patty was admitted on a Monday for routine preoperative tests to be followed by surgery on Thursday. Those were three very tense days for all of us, as the suspicion began to grow that, when the given day came, Krane would not be able to find his valvulotome, the specially designed knifelike instrument that cuts the stenotic valve open and allows normal blood flow. Krane had done this relatively new operation several times before, but always on adolescents, whose lesser degree of stenosis had allowed them to live longer and therefore presented a significantly smaller risk.

During outpatient visits and the three preoperative days in the hospital, I had gotten to know the Crawfords quite well. Jack was an accountant for a small sales firm, and Gwen had been a bookkeeper before she married him and then gave birth to Patty's only sibling, a perfectly healthy girl named Nancy, two years before Patty's arrival. Both Jack and Gwen were kind and understanding people and, like the families of most of Krane's patients, admired him. And why not? He was a soft-spoken, gentle man whose quiet though firm South Carolina accent instilled confidence, especially in people who had absolutely no idea how nervous and even agitated he could sometimes become in the operating room. Like all the other members of Krane's team, I had become very fond of my little patient's parents.

It was Krane's habit to have two of his assistant residents bring every one of his patients to the OR on the morning of surgery, rather than trusting even such a routine assignment to orderlies. And so it came to be that Ken Stettman and I wheeled Patty directly into the scene of chaos taking place outside Room #3, which Krane used on alternate days with Cannon. As predicted by so many of us, the valvulotome was missing. Just as predictably, Jim Hartenberg, the chief of pediatric cardiology, was beside himself with anger. He had been through so many of Krane's subterfuges that this one was too obvious to look like anything but the fraud that it actually was.

Hartenberg knew Krane much better than the rest of us did. The two had served at the same naval hospital during World War II, and were close contemporaries and even friends. Hartenberg had long become inured to Krane's hesitancy on any given morning, but he was determined that this was not to be one of those days. He very well knew that should Patty not have her operation very soon, she would never have it: His otherwise much-admired friend would not be able to work up the courage anytime within the next six months, which was Hartenberg's estimated time for her continuing survival.

So, as we were all being dispersed to the usual places to seek the missing valvulotome, Hartenberg wasted no time. Having previously arranged for Krane to receive an urgent call to come to Cannon's office at precisely this moment, he hurried down to the office of the cardiac surgeon. Opening the top middle drawer of Krane's desk, he picked up the valvulotome and slowly ascended the three flights of stairs to the OR, giving his colleague enough time to return from his wild goose chase. As Krane reached him, Hartenberg slapped the small instrument into the reluctant surgeon's palm and said, loudly enough for the head nurse to hear, "Now go operate."

Krane blushed deeply, mumbled a few inaudible words, and ordered that Patty's gurney be wheeled from the corridor into the OR. To the uncomprehending little girl herself, he gave a broad smile of deep confidence and said, "We're gonna fix you up good as new, honey," and then walked resolutely off toward the scrub room.

Four hours later, Ken and I wheeled Patty to the recovery room. Functioning normally inside her chest was a wide-open pulmonary valve. She would grow up to become a lawyer in Milwaukee, have three healthy children of her own, and revere Richard Custis Krane, the brave surgeon who had saved her life.

As for Krane and Hartenberg, five years later one of the major pediatric journals published their article about the longest successful series of pulmonary valvulotomies in children under the age of ten, all done with the instrument so conveniently found that morning in the top middle drawer of the surgeon's desk.

CR

The Anesthesiologist's Tale

NESTHESIOLOGISTS LOVE TO TELL stories about surgeons, and I have my share of them. After twenty-five
years of putting people to sleep, I thought I had seen
just about everything, good and bad. But the Tale I'm about to
relate is in a category of its own, and I doubt that anyone but the
people present in the operating room that day could tell its like.
Or at least, I hope not.

I've discussed this case with colleagues in anesthesia and surgery, malpractice lawyers, forensic psychiatrists, and anyone else
who might have heard of such a horrendous thing, and, other
than those who were actually there with me to witness the event,

none have experienced anything comparable. I don't doubt that such situations may have occurred in eras long gone by, but in those days they were hardly intended for the healing of the man or woman subjected to them. And though there is no evidence of it, who knows but that one or two of the so-called Nazi Doctors may have been guilty of the kind of thing about which you are about to read? One forensic shrink did tell me of a vague recollection from his medical school days, but he wasn't able to document any of its facts.

Now and then, one picks up a newspaper and reads of a maniac who has murdered and brutalized the bodies of any number of men, women, and children, but the details are so grim that the average reader is repelled by them, and in any event, here too, healing is not the intent.

Two and a half millennia ago, the Hippocratic physicians of Greece taught their successors—us—the simple dictum that the duty of the healer is "to do good, or at least to do no harm," which was later Latinized to the oft-quoted *primum non nocere,* do no harm. Hardly a doctor lives who has not on more than one occasion quoted that aphorism, and all of us attempt to live by it. Not only do we live by it, but we establish principles of ethics and morals so strictly distinctive that we do whatever is possible to keep others of our medical brethren from breaching it.

Ethicists debate the level of responsibility that any individual physician has in monitoring his or her professional colleagues, but no one questions that to look over another's shoulder is a good thing. It is not only a moral responsibility, but a community one, too, that gave rise to the many hospital committees that oversee one or another aspect of the dealings between the healers and those who come to them for healing. Furthermore, lay members of institutional boards were keeping a close eye on doctors long before anyone had ever heard the term "bioethics." For all of these reasons, those associated with the art of healing assume a personal responsibility when they take on the more general one of being part of the community they have chosen for their life's work. We are indeed our brothers' keepers, which is one of the reasons that I felt personally compelled to choose this Tale when asked to describe my most memorable patient.

My story begins in a way that would seem to contradict some of the high-minded rhetoric you have just read. I have been describing all patients as being our joint responsibility, and now will proceed to tell of this particular one as though he were the patient of one doctor only—and that doctor was not, in fact, me. This, of course, is one of the paradoxes of being an anesthesiologist: A surgical patient comes into the hospital for an operation, not an anesthetic; he is referred to by everyone connected with him as the patient of a particular surgeon, and yet we who provide the surgical sleep consider him our charge. We review his records, examine him, speak to consultants who may be involved in his care, often meet with family members before the operation, and in other ways think of him as *our* patient. One of our most important responsibilities is to protect him from the metabolic and physiologic stresses to which the surgery must necessarily expose him.

And so, should something go amiss during the procedure, though it has nothing to do with our specific role in the entire course of events, we carefully review what we might have done to prevent it. But every once in a while, a complication of such an unusual nature takes place that we are left only with a sense of guilt, though careful review of each of our actions reveals not a single obvious error that we should have avoided or a difficulty we should have been able to predict. On the other hand, an anesthesiologist is sometimes as culpable as though he had committed the error with his own fingers and mind.

With this long prelude involving morals on the one hand and mayhem on the other—plus a few comments on the uniqueness of what is to be described—you are, I hope, prepared to read a story like no other, which I have already claimed this Tale to be. Yes, the patient was mine in each sense I have described; though in the eyes of the community—hospital and otherwise—he was the responsibility of the surgeon, Bill Mansfield, in my own eyes there will always remain the image of a man who almost died while I looked on, and therefore a profound portrait of guilt. The guilt persists, and even grows, because though I have reviewed every aspect of the near-tragedy again and again, I always come away with the puzzle of why I behaved as passively as I did.

I had known Bill Mansfield long before he was aware of my existence. He had been an all-star fullback on my high school football team during the year I was a freshman. Though we both went on to the same college—where he captained the varsity and I played in the marching band—and medical school, our paths rarely crossed, so I thought of him as an acquaintance rather than as a friend or close colleague.

Physically, Bill was one helluva large guy. At six foot three and some 250 pounds, he looked the part of a surgeon, though one might more likely have mistaken him for an orthopedist than a specialist in the area he chose, the abdomen and entire field of what was then called general surgery. Someone his size is expected to be rather louder and perhaps more demanding than most, but Bill surprised people by his quiet demeanor and general sense of decorum in the operating room. By all accounts, no one had ever heard him use the occasional foul language to which his colleagues were sometime prone when things were not going to their liking during a case. He was known to be especially courteous to the nurses, another trait that surgeons sometimes forgo or forget in the heat of battle. And to women doctors like me, he was the soul of all that we ask for: dignity and the sense of total equality. Though he and I rarely did an operation together (my particular interest is in cardiac anesthesia, and I work in general surgery only on days when there is no heart to repair), I always looked forward to those unusual occasions when I saw his name listed for a patient whose anesthetic I was to give. I was hardly alone among my fellow department members in this regard, because he seemed to have a fine respect for the role we play in the management of the operation—this, too, not being a particularly common characteristic among his cutting colleagues.

As far as I could tell, Bill had only one problem. Though hardly a secret, it was rarely the subject of conversation among his peers, because to speak of it would be like gossiping against a man highly respected: He had some sort of psychiatric condition, for which he required medication whose nature was not known to anyone except the chief of surgery, to whom his psychiatrist was required to submit a status report once each month. Because of his quiet demeanor, I had always assumed that it was a mild chronic depression that had no effect on the fine quality of his operating room methods or patient care.

No one had ever reported any irregularity in Bill's work. Quite to the contrary, his technique and timing were so predictable that it was sometimes said of him that he'd finish any routine case within ten minutes of the time it had taken him to do the previous one of the same sort. This was a rare trait in a surgeon and much appreciated by everyone on the staff. We did, after all, need to not only fulfill our routine daily schedule but leave sufficient time for add-ons, whether urgent or emergent. To have one or two men like Bill on the surgical service made everything easier for all of us. In fact, it had been reported at the community hospital where Bill often worked that he had several years earlier done four consecutive splenectomies for Hodgkin's disease in a single day when that operation was at its height of popularity, and finished each one in seventy-five to eighty-five minutes, neither more nor less.

What I am trying to convey here is the absolute steadiness of the man. He had three children between the ages of twelve and twenty-one almost exactly three years apart; owned a typical suburban house with a two-Volvo garage alongside it; took a three-week vacation each year, always going to the same Caribbean island; and voted Republican in every election from President to town council. In fact, he had been a town councilman himself, serving his community with distinction for some five terms of two years each, and, had he not been a surgeon, would certainly have been considered an ideal candidate for mayor or state senator.

Bill had what might be called a medium-sized practice; he kept his roster of cases at a particular level from year to year. Because he did about half of his operating at the community hospital across town, I'd see him in our OR no more frequently than every two or three days. So it was with some anticipation on a lovely February afternoon in 1985 that I saw his name on my own schedule for the following morning for what was to be a routine cholecystectomy, removal of the gallbladder. In his hands, such a procedure would almost certainly take between forty-five and fifty minutes, allowing us to fill out the rest of our day with the two hernias and a thyroid that were to follow in succession.

The patient, Morton Cantrell, was a perfectly healthy— though obese—fifty-five-year-old accountant who had been without symptoms until about two months earlier, when he'd had his first and only attack of nausea and upper abdominal pain shortly after eating a particularly fatty meal at a downtown retail conference. In his usual thorough leave-nothing-to-chance way, Mansfield had worked him up as an outpatient, found a few small stones, and recommended operation. Cantrell had chosen our hospital rather than the bigger community hospital because it was closer to his home and easier for his wife to visit. In those days, even a gallbladder operation meant a stay of about seven days, so the difference in distance had some importance.

One of the OR secretaries the morning of surgery had commented to the head nurse of my room that the ordinarily stolid but unfailingly courteous Professor Mansfield seemed in a particularly jolly mood as he entered the doctors' locker room at 7:30 A.M., an unusual situation she attributed to that day being his first back at work after his yearly vacation. I was already in the room busying myself with inserting Mr. Cantrell's intravenous line, so I didn't give her remark much thought until the surgeon himself entered, obviously in the sort of overtly gregarious mood in which I had never seen him. Ignoring my warm greeting on his return, he ignored his patient as well, another first in my experience of him. Instead, he stepped forward and fondled the left breast of the unscrubbed head nurse and planted a noisy kiss on her forehead. She was so shocked, and even frazzled, that not a single word issued from a mouth that ordinarily would have given a full dressing-down to anyone else who had done such an outrageous thing. But this was, after all, Dr. Mansfield, and she may have thought that if such a sedate, well-mannered surgeon had behaved this way, there must have been something about herself that had provoked it, an emotion well known to women who have just been badly treated by men from whom they had good reason to expect better. So Mansfield got away not only with his bad behavior, but also with a very short but very dirty joke he told as he disappeared into the scrub room.

The surgeon was back in less than half the time it takes to do a ten-minute scrub and told yet another story of the same sort, seeming surprised when one of the technicians protested that he seemed hardly himself. By this time, Cantrell was asleep and intubated, the assisting intern had put the drapes in place, and Mansfield—to everyone's unbelieving horror—began operating as though in a world gone mad. He was in Cantrell's obese belly within about a minute, had the gall bladder out in two or three minutes more, and was beginning to dissect the stomach, not bothering to tie off any but the largest vessels, leaving the smaller ones to spurt bright red arterial blood onto the drapes and over the masks of the assistants. Before I realized how far he'd gone, he tossed that perfectly normal section of stomach into a specimen pan and—right before our astonished eyes—cut a transverse slash through the front wall of the aorta. The decibel level in the room rose as high as the column of blood blasting its lethal way toward the ceiling, and in moments the room was filled with everyone who was within sound of it. An orderly even bigger than Mansfield himself grabbed him from behind, wrestled his huge bulk away from the table, and pinned him to the floor, all while the obviously crazed surgeon was yelling, "What the hell do you think you're doing, boy?" and then, "This is a sterile field you've just contaminated, you dumb asshole!"

Meanwhile, the quick-handed intern had managed to ram a large sponge onto the front of the hemorrhaging aorta, applying enough pressure to slow the bleeding considerably. The uproarious din emanating from the room was heard by two of our vascular surgeons down the corridor waiting for their case to start, and they immediately were gowned and gloved without wasting precious time scrubbing. Their sterile kit of specialized instruments was rolled in, and they had the aorta stitched and completely repaired in ten minutes. A team of general surgeons reattached the mangled torn ends of the stomach, and by the time they were through with their reconstructive tailoring, a reasonable facsimile of its original had been made, though a great deal smaller. I had called for universal-donor blood and was pumping as hard as I could until the patient's blood pressure, which had been immeasurable at the height of the crisis, reappeared and reached a relatively normal level. During all of this, Mansfield, almost completely hidden under three orderlies, was threatening to sue all of us.

It was Cantrell, of course, who did the suing. When I later read the full list of defendants, it appeared as though his team of lawyers had named everyone within a mile of the hospital and collected from more than half a dozen. Needless to say, one of them was me. Other than Mansfield himself—who lost not only the lawsuits but his license to practice medicine (and almost his freedom)—the biggest losers were the chiefs of surgery at the two hospitals where the doctor whom the local newspapers soon dubbed "The Wild Man of Borneo" did his operating. Their supervision, declared the final court papers, was "negligent to the point of being outrageously so." Both lost their jobs.

In the unlikely event that you've not already guessed it, Bill Mansfield's "some sort of psychiatric condition" was bipolar disorder, and he had been off his medications for the entire length of his three-week family vacation. He had never previously violated the terms of his psychiatric supervision, with the result that no one had thought to have his medication levels tested before allowing him back into the OR following his return. William Rogers Mansfield was the most reliable of men, and why should anyone doubt what was universally called his predictability? Even his wife of twenty-five years had not known of the "experiment," as he called it in court, that he had decided to conduct on himself during the family's time on St. Thomas, though she did mention at one of the hearings that his sexual needs seemed to have magnified during the final week.

And as for Cantrell, he may have ended up being the biggest winner of all, and not only in respect to money. To begin with, he had his gallbladder taken out gratis and became a multimillionaire at the same time. The decrease in the size of his stomach anticipated by about fifteen years a somewhat similar modern procedure called a surgical stapling, so he is nowadays a svelte figure of a seventy-five-year-old man. The previously healthy aorta repaired is still a perfectly healthy aorta, so that specific part of his huge operation, though potentially the most life-threatening at the time it was done, has affected his daily doings not a bit. And for all of the mayhem and failures of sterility in the OR on that most memorable of mornings, he developed not a single postoperative complication. And Morton Cantrell is grateful for something else as well: He never had to work another day in his life.

಼

Commentary to
The Anesthesiologist's Tale

As Karishma Noticewala, the anesthesiologist of this Tale, points out, healing the sick has become a joint responsibility, especially in today's large medical centers where the great majority of those involved in care are completely unknown to the patient, who may never so much as lay eyes on them. Most patients are probably aware of the necessity of this situation, but it is also true that very few hospitalized men and women have any idea of how seriously most staff members—at least those professionally trained—treat the charge that defines their responsibilities. But it is precisely that notion—the definition of responsibility—that Karishma grapples with, as do all anesthesiologists.

Much of this has to do with the history of the specialty. It is hardly an exaggeration to say that it took an entire century for anesthesiologists to become full partners in the endeavor called an operation. From the first use of ether at the Massachusetts General Hospital on October 16, 1846, until the early 1950s, far too little was known about the abstruse details of the body's response to an anesthetic. It was only in the 1950s that certain pioneers in a very few academic centers began to unravel the hormonal, cardiopulmonary, neuromuscular, and other implications of what would seem to be the simple technical performance of putting even the healthiest of patients to sleep. As Karishma states very clearly, "a surgical patient comes into the hospital for an operation, not an anesthetic," and yet the outcome of that operation may have less to do with the skill and watchfulness of the person holding the knife than of the one who is administering the vapors of Morpheus.

Karishma's soul-searching of that ultimate truth began during her residency days, long before the Mansfield–Cantrell fiasco. But since that event, she has developed a more all-inclusive viewpoint, one that makes her as much an expert on surveillance as she is on sleep. She is convinced that Mansfield's mayhem was her fault; she is convinced that the malpractice judgment against her was correct. And if you'd like my own opinion, I am convinced that she is right.

"To do no harm" also must be understood as "to allow no harm," and that is the precept that Karishma violated. Mansfield's first moment in the operating room should have alerted her that something was amiss in the behavior of this man of steady habits. Karishma is aware of this, talks about it, and exhibits a valuable kind of courage by telling the Tale exactly as it occurred, so that a reader of even the least subtle form of mind can easily see her role in the circumstances. To Karishma Noticewala, Mansfield was no more guilty than she herself, and she wants that known.

Many decades ago when I was in surgical training, we occasionally debated the "captain of the ship" concept. Is the captain the surgeon, the internist, the patient's own referring physician, or the anesthesiologist? Who, indeed, should have the final word on decisions? In those days, what we were debating was authority. Far more important to the patient's welfare is responsibility, and it belongs to all of us who would call ourselves healers.

⚘

The Neurosurgeon's Tale(s)

BEFORE LAUNCHING INTO MY Tale, I'd like to tell a much shorter one, just to give some idea of a dictum of mine. Of course, the dictum applies to all medicine, but it seems to work itself out more commonly in my specialty of pediatric neurosurgery than in most others: "I see and treat a lot of ferocious problems—trauma, congenital anomalies, tumors. In my business, you can lose big, but sometimes you win big, too."

Let me get the bad stuff over with, as briefly as I can. This first story is about a two-and-a-half-year-old boy whom we had to rush directly to the operating room from the emergency room late one night with a ghastly injury to his head, later revealed to have been caused by his mother's boyfriend—by every description a monstrous hulk of inhumanity—who had thrown the child against the wall in a fit of rage, with all the strength his six feet and some 200 pounds could inflict. The boy's body was covered in bruises, most of which were days old, and his body temperature was far subnormal. But as horrifying as was all of this, the most heartrending injury was an extensive tear in the rectum, about the origin of which none of us wanted to conjecture, at least not out loud.

The injury to the little boy's brain was so extensive and the bleeding so profuse that nothing could be done, despite efforts by the entire operating room crew that I can only call heroic. I haven't had many children die in the OR, so I rarely witness the kind of sorrow I saw that night—were this at all a common experience, no one in the world could be induced to choose such a specialty. One of the nurses, who I later learned had a little boy exactly this kid's age, was working through a screen of tears as we desperately tried to stop the unremitting tide of bleeding from deep within the brain's substance. When it was all over, the scene of carnage became a scene of grief, or perhaps "lamentation" is a better word to describe the raw emotion and the sounds of anguish filling the room, and not only from the women. I've seen worse head injuries, but I've never seen a more abused child, and I've never left an operating room so heartsick.

Certain kinds of statements are never to be written in a patient's chart. But on this one night, I seem to have lost control of any pretence of restraint. I was beyond caring what my words would look like should they ever be read aloud in a courtroom, which, in fact, they eventually were. All through the hectic moments in the OR, the police had been holding my little patient's mother under arrest in a small cubicle of the emergency room. Because as the chief surgeon I could not shirk my responsibility for telling her of the child's death, it became my distasteful obligation to see her, face to face. But I had not expected the murderous brute to be there as well. The officers had easily tracked him down, and one of them stood there with a drawn revolver aimed at his head, a sight I had never expected to see in a hospital. But I'm sure I would have done the same had I been in the cop's shoes.

I uttered only a brief sentence to the mother—"Kevin is dead"—and I was able to get it out of my mouth as though without emotion. But then I could not help turning to the behemoth and positioning myself on a chair so that my face was within inches of his bloodshot and now terrified eyes. I wanted to be sure that he could see the bits of brain clinging to my OR gown, the front of which was soaked in the fresh still-scarlet blood of the child he had killed. "This is what you did," was all I was able to say, because I was afraid I'd vomit if I tried to speak another word.

I stood up and went back upstairs to the OR, where the intern was writing his operative note in the chart. I waited patiently until he was finished, then took his pen and printed clearly, so there would be no misreading it at some future date, "The mother and her boyfriend are the stuff of worst nightmares." I signed my name in letters larger than usual, and walked toward the surgeons' shower room to try somehow to wash away what I had seen that night.

BUT "SOMETIMES YOU WIN big, too," and this next Tale is of one of those victories. Words like "win" and "victory" are relative in my specialty, and not every reader of this story might agree that matters turned out as one's fondest hopes might have fantasized. But they did indeed turn out very well nevertheless. And it is for this reason that I consider Maryann Dugan the most memorable patient I have ever seen.

I first met Maryann before she was born, when one of the obstetricians asked me to see a twenty-nine-year-old woman whose child, due for delivery in only a few weeks, had been diagnosed with massive hydrocephalus. This takes some explaining. Within the brain are four spaces—known as ventricles—of various sizes and shapes, communicating with each other and with the canal running up the center of the spinal cord. Membranes lining the ventricles produce what is called cerebrospinal fluid, which circulates among the ventricles, brain, and cord, bathing and bringing essential nutrients to the tissues. Should some obstruction occur during embryonic development, the fluid cannot move freely, resulting in its accumulation throughout the interconnecting system, with enlargement of the ventricles, pressure on the brain, and an increase in the size of the head. This is the condition commonly called water on the brain.

At the time I met Maryann in utero, the only effective treatment for hydrocephalus was to insert a valved, plastic tube into one of the ventricles, bring it out through a small hole in the skull, and pass it into the abdomen, tunneling a pathway just beneath the skin. This way, the excess fluid empties into the abdominal cavity and the pressure on the brain is relieved. When the condition is not severe and is diagnosed early, it is possible for a child to live an entirely normal life. But that is not always the case, and some children are left with mental defects of various degree.

Maryann's parents had been looking forward to the pregnancy for about two years. They had been shown the ultrasound, so I was able to speak with complete frankness about the size of the baby's head. To my surprise, their acceptance of the situation was remarkable, especially considering the likelihood that there might be some significant brain damage even with placement of the shunt within hours of delivery.

A cesarean section was scheduled, and as soon as it was completed I hurried over to the Newborn Special Care unit to greet my new patient, prepared to take her directly to the operating room. On the way I met the family, just out of the delivery room with the mother holding her new baby happily in her arms, and the father beaming with pride as though he were looking not at a child with an adult-sized head, but at the perfect baby everyone hopes for. I had never seen a larger skull in a newborn, but the parents were oblivious to its size. All they could think about was their happiness, wanting to share it with me, though I was almost a complete stranger to them.

Throughout her entire life, these two devoted people have treated Maryann exactly as they were doing at that moment. They never had another child—everything in their hearts was showered on this little girl born with such a serious defect that her survival itself was doubtful for weeks, until all the complexities of the necessary surgery were completed and her recovery became likely. Not only did she require a shunt, but the plastic surgeons and I had to carry out a series of intricate procedures in order to reduce the size of her skull to more normal proportions as the hydrocephalus decreased.

Maryann's intellectual development was slow at first, but within time she began to approximate her peers, though she never did quite catch up until well into adolescence—and even then her progress was largely due to the encouragement she received from her extraordinary parents. There were problems along the way, as there so often are in children with congenital hydrocephalus: She has had seizures; her shunt has needed to be revised on several occasions, though successfully each time; she developed an infection in the tubing when the family was on vacation more than two thousand miles away, and had to be rushed back to Canterbury in time for effective treatment.

Yet as wonderful as her parents have been, the real wonder is Maryann herself, a lovely, self-confident young woman who is now a twenty-year-old college sophomore. When she was about ten, I asked that she come to the annual lecture I give to our medical students on hydrocephalus. It was the first of several visits she made, and I remember well the bounce in her blond, braided hair as she skipped up and down the stairs of the large lecture hall, chatting up one student after another. And there was the famous clinic visit that our nurses still talk about. For years, I've given a quarter to each child who comes to see me in follow-up. On this particular visit, Maryann arrived carrying an entire bag of collected quarters she'd been saving to share with the other kids.

There was another big win to this Tale, beyond the victory of a little girl with a charming personality who overcame massive odds to become an exemplar of what can sometimes be accomplished when the will and the support are so strong. Enter once again Maryann's parents, Frank and Peggy Dugan. In later years the Dugans achieved great success in what had begun as a small cardboard-box business opened a few years after their daughter's birth. In her name, they established an entirely new department in a small college devoted to teaching young adults who need a lot of extra help in order to live independently in a complex world.

୧୭

Commentary to *The Neurosurgeon's Tale(s)*

Like many neurosurgeons, Forrest Harrison cultivates an air—no, call it an aura—of remote superiority. Depending on how well one knows the men, and more recently the women, who have populated this demanding specialty, the aura may be seen as either a genuine cloak of aloofness intended to intimidate colleagues in other fields of medicine or a carapace of well-disguised protection against the hurts they encounter in their everyday activities. The contents of the skull and spinal column permit few errors, and the smallest hint of fallibility tempts frail tissue toward revenge.

The specialty as we know it today was founded shortly after the turn of the twentieth century by Harvey Cushing, a young Johns Hopkins surgeon with talents enough to man an entire department, and then some. Confronted by the risky mysteries of cerebral function and intrigued by the difficulties of approaching the brain's anatomy with even a modicum of safety, he set himself the task of learning as much as he could about the tapioca-textured organ that has mystified since the art of healing first began, and probably long before that as well.

As he gradually came to develop techniques allowing reasonably safe approaches to brain and nerve tissue, Cushing gathered around him a group of men very much like himself in personality, though it would be impossible to approach emulating that unique combination of inborn and carefully cultivated talents that elevated him above almost every other surgeon of his time. Like their chief, they were tough enough to take on challenges few others would dare face, and—equally like him—they held themselves at a far remove from those they considered less able to withstand the enormously long hours under constant technical and psychic tension necessary to accomplish critical objectives. With few exceptions, that first generation of Cushing disciples were not nice men. In the name of the arcane art they were developing, a wake of considerable rancor was left, which took their successors great effort to dissipate.

Several generations have passed since that time, and the image of the neurosurgeon has finally softened. But that does not mean that either the cloak or the carapace is no longer worn. Both retain their traditional uses, and the attentive skill of a thoughtful observer lies in telling one from the other, or any intermediate material being used to cover the truth dwelling inside.

Though I was in no clinical contact with him, I had, for years, assumed Forrest Harrison to be a true, undiluted descendant of Harvey Cushing. Having served on a few hospital committees together, our acquaintance was superficial except during a few brief periods when we worked with small groups sharing administrative interests. What I observed was a deceptively soft-spoken North Carolinian who loved a good fight, especially if, as often happened, he found himself the only representative of a particularly contentious point of view opposed by some hospital administrator. With just a hint of menacing snarl sometimes detectable, the pitch of those otherwise dulcet tones would on occasion become harsh. In an instant he'd be riding into battle on a figurative white charger, as though brandishing a tide of resentment for having lost a long-ago war that would have been won had virtue been the deciding factor rather than numbers (that, of course, may only have been my impression). And then the softness would return as quickly as it had disappeared, though leaving behind not only the impression that he cared not a whit whom he had offended, but also elements of a whirlwind waiting to be released if needed. Harrison shared with the rest of us a deep interest in excellence of patient care, but seemed often to differ on just how best to provide it. He never left his competition with a hint of compromise or even a suggestion that anyone—especially an administrator—knew how to solve problems except himself. When the occasion demanded, he was one tough guy in the Harvey Cushing mode, with only the Carolinian drawl to distinguish him from his professional forebear. In short, he was unrecognizable at those conferences as the Forrest Harrison whose Tales you have just read.

I learned of the real man on a single August evening twenty-three years ago, and thereon hangs another Tale. My fourth child, Sally, was born with a slightly enlarged skull, but no one—not even her surgeon father—thought much of it. Her kindly, avuncular pediatrician, Albert Pious, considered her perfectly normal and her early development singularly unremarkable. In fact, her large skull became a bit of a joke in the family, being compared to that of a well-loved maternal uncle. That she might have an abnormality never occurred to any of us.

Fortunately for the conclusion of this Tale, Sally developed a widespread rash on her right thigh one evening when she was three months old, and her mother took her to the pediatrician the following afternoon. Having completed the day's operating schedule, I entered my office at about 2:00 P.M. to begin seeing the afternoon's round of patients. No sooner had I put on a white coat than my longtime assistant, Annie Gambardella, told me that I was wanted on the phone by Chris Cutler, who was covering for the vacationing Pious. For reasons that only the unconscious mind will ever be able to explain, I was thunderstruck. Something deep inside a compartment of the brain that may exist only in a psychoanalyst's obscure theory instantly said, "Of course—he's going to tell me that my child has hydrocephalus," a thought that had not entered my consciousness until that very fraction of a millisecond. It was as though some part of my deepest awareness had always known, but stubbornly refused to acknowledge it. The first words out of Chris's mouth confirmed that I—or that place so deep inside—was right.

I dashed the three flights up to Pious's office, where my wife, Kate, was preparing to take Sally down to the radiology department for an ultrasound of her head. The study showed mild but unmistakable evidence of hydrocephalus. As gently as he could, Chris pointed out that a bit of bulging of the child's eyes was already beginning to make itself evident, and no time was to be lost—a pediatric neurosurgeon had to be consulted immediately. He recommended Harrison, but my previous contacts with that meteoric worthy had left me with an image so Cushingesque that I spent a few wasted hours—four, if it can be believed, so great was my antipathy to that quietly aggressive personality—trying to locate another surgeon, with whom I had trained. It turned out that he was on a sailboat somewhere and unreachable, but it took all that time to be sure.

Meanwhile, Kate had taken Sally to the emergency room after finally giving up on the other surgeon, and I agreed with some reluctance to let the neurosurgical resident call Harrison. By then it was early evening, but Harrison arrived only half an hour later, strolling into the ER cubicle as though on his laconic way to a first predinner cocktail. As always, though, his seemingly lackadaisical movements belied the lightning speed of his mind. He greeted both of us with surprising warmth, and then turned every bit of his prodigious ability to concentrate on our little Sally, cooing at her as though at play while he tested her reflexes and meticulously carried out every bit of a complete neurological examination. When he had unhurriedly finished every element of his exam—which, in our anxiety, seemed to take hours—he looked up with a kindness of which I'd not considered him capable. "Yes," he drawled as slowly as I had ever heard him speak, "Sally does have hydrocephalus." One remembers small things from such moments, and how well I recall the long seconds he left between his first sentence and the second. "It's a bit farther advanced than I'd like, so we'll put in a shunt first thing in the morning. Meantime, we'll transfer her to the Pediatric Intensive Care Unit for the night, just so we can watch her more carefully."

With that, he did something unforgettable, as though he knew exactly what the art of medicine demanded at that moment and has demanded since Hippocrates first articulated such things. As Kate cradled Sally in her lap, Harrison put his arm around my shoulder and slowly walked me out of the room, explaining as softly and encouragingly as he could that he expected my baby to do well. That I was a dozen years his senior and a full academic rank above him was not a consideration at that moment—to him, I was a worried father, and I needed the reassurance that could only come from him. I knew that I was putting my trust not in the hotshot neurosurgeon about to perform some wondrous feat—though all of this was true—but in the hands and mind of a kind, capable physician, who would do all in his power to bring my baby, and her parents, safely through the ordeal they were about to face.

Sally did indeed do well. For twenty-one years she was without any difficulty, but then required a complex revision of her shunt from which she finally recovered after a series of several hazardous operations. But she is a healthy and perfectly normal young woman today, still adores Forrest Harrison, and sees him as we do, and as do all of his patients, his assistants, and the grateful parents to whom he has always brought all the reassurance of which he is so abundantly capable: To them, he is the empathic man who wrote the two Neurosurgeon's Tales.

The Chest Surgeon's Tale(s)

M Y TALE HAS TWO parts, and they bear no relationship to each other. I reserve this privilege on the basis of seniority: I am a real antique now, about ten years older than any of the other physicians in this book, and what is most memorable to me are several moments during my training years in the post–World War II period when I took part in an adventure or two that I find unforgettable.

Only one of them involved a patient. He was deeply anesthetized at the time and never knew how memorable he would become—memorable, that is, because of something I did, but in which he was a totally passive participant. While the other story I've chosen to tell is a Tale having nothing to do with any patient, it certainly does illustrate how different things were in those times than they are now, and how we (or at least I) sometimes used to get away with bad behavior by using a combination of quick-wittedness and even more bad behavior. That Tale doesn't belong in this book—or probably in any book for that matter—but the Narrator has let me tell it in order to humor me in my dotage. It doesn't reflect well on me, but we made a bargain. If he wanted the first Tale, he had to take the second along with it.

First things first. The year was 1947, and I had just returned from three years in the Army Medical Corps. My intention had been to train in chest surgery, and what better place to find myself after discharge than back at Canterbury Hospital? The chief of the Thoracic Section was the fabled Carl Swenson, and he seemed to know everything. Not only that, but he had a burning desire to teach. He had spent two years in the navy near the end of the war, as one of only a few surgeons well qualified to operate on the lungs and esophagus, with the result that his clinical experience was vast.

Swenson enjoyed nothing more than taking one of his trainees through some difficult procedure, and I was the beneficiary of his enthusiasm. My own experience during the three years in the army while in Europe had also been extensive, so I had come to Canterbury to put the finishing touches on what I already considered a high degree of proficiency.

I carefully chose the cases in which I wanted to partici-pate, being sure to select those that I, or the professor, thought most challenging. But when not actually operating or caring for patients on the wards, I enjoyed watching Swenson work, so I would often come up to his special room in OR #3 and stand on a low stool across from him as he demonstrated operating on a tumor, an unusual anatomical malformation, or some similar structure not often seen.

This Tale took place one morning when the chief was operating on a fourteen-year-old boy with a vascular condition called patent ductus arteriosus. The ductus, as I'll call it from here on, is a short artery whose purpose during prenatal life is to allow blood to bypass the lungs, which are not yet functioning. The vessel almost always closes soon after birth, allowing the normal circulation that permits proper flow to each of the two lungs as they fill with air. But every once in a great while a ductus stays open, allowing too much blood to enter the lung tissue under high pressure. Symptoms are usually minimal for years, but too long a period of such an excess may cause difficulty, so it is almost always recommended that the ductus be tied off or divided, a relatively safe procedure pioneered in the early 1940s as one of the first operations done on vessels involving the circulation of the lungs or heart. Needless to say, Carl Swenson was an expert at the procedure, and even I had done a few.

The most impressive characteristic of a patent ductus is a murmur so harsh that it sounds through the stethoscope like a machinery shop running at full blast. In fact, the rush of blood through the short length of vessel creates such a tumult through the chest wall that it can often be felt with the examining doctor's hand placed just to the left of the upper part of the breastbone, a phenomenon called a thrill because of its vibratory quality.

The boy being operated upon that day demonstrated all the characteristics of a typical ductus, except that his thrill was particularly difficult to feel during the admitting examination. When Swenson had the vessel cleanly dissected and exposed, he instructed the junior resident, Pete Curtis, to place his gloved finger on its surface so that he might confirm that the thrill was actually present. But no matter how hard he tried, whether with great delicacy or firm pressure, Pete could not convince himself that the vibration was coming through to his satisfaction. Guided by Swenson, he twisted his hand every which way, always to no avail.

The temptation was too much for me. There I was, all six feet three inches and 140 pounds of experienced and perhaps over-enthusiastic surgeon hovering ever closer over the operative field, unable to avoid the inevitable—to which I finally succumbed. With both skinny arms extended into the chest cavity, I bent the final two inches forward, took the ductus into one bare hand, and twisted it just a bit between thumb and first finger, hearing myself say in a clear, altogether too loud, voice, "What the hell is the matter with you, Curtis? Hold the fucking thing in just that way and you can't miss feeling that damn thrill."

The room fell dead silent. Realizing what I had done—not to mention the salty army language accompanying it—I jerked my hands out of the chest, almost falling backward off the stool as I straightened my body to an upright position. Too late. Swenson stared up at me with horror and even a look of hate in his blazing blue eyes. And then he did something unimaginable—even more unimaginable than my having violated a sterile field with ungloved hands: He threw the largest hemostatic clamp within reach, right into my face. Without a moment's hesitation, he then ran around the foot of the table and began to chase me. Fortunately, he was much shorter than I, and a bit awkward in the legs. But I dissipated the lead I had gotten on him by stepping down from the observation stool without looking, with the result that my size-twelve left foot squeezed itself tightly into an adjoining sponge pail.

Even now, sixty years later, I have trouble believing that this scene was really taking place. There I was, pail and all, stomping toward the double doors of Room #3, with the infuriated (beware the wrath of the Norsemen, the Celts used to say, when they saw those threatening longboats on the horizon) Swenson chasing me as fast as his closely encompassing surgical gown allowed. Luckily for me, he tripped on an extension tube of the anesthesia apparatus and lost his balance for a moment, but he quickly regained it and resumed pursuit. But by this time, I had shaken my foot loose of the sponge pail and had a substantial lead. The last words I heard from my chief—and to this day they still ring in my ears—were: "And don't you ever try to come back, at least while I'm alive!"

And that's how I lost my job at Canterbury. Fortunately for me, a teaching hospital in northern Michigan had just lost their chief resident, who had come down with a fresh case of tuberculosis, not an uncommon situation in those days. Desperate for a replacement and despite a harsh letter from Swenson, they took me on, enabling me to complete my formal training and qualify as a chest surgeon.

But the Tale doesn't end there. Twenty years later, by then a professor myself at a reasonably good university hospital, I was asked to introduce Carl Swenson's valedictory at the end of a retirement dinner in his honor, held at a Chicago meeting of the American College of Surgeons. I had had no communication with him during all those years, but I delivered the usual flowery encomium, of course, not daring to mention my bare-handed grab of that ductus two decades earlier. The old chief, perhaps because he was by that point virtually embalmed with aquavit, thanked me graciously for my kind words. But he couldn't keep himself from adding, as the final sentence of his brief remarks, the comment that "Should Dr. Catledge still be wondering, the young man whose ductus he may recall fondling one day at Canterbury had a very smooth postoperative course. I'm glad to see that Catledge himself recovered as well."

THE NARRATOR WILL PROBABLY tell you that I'm a scoundrel, but I've always had a perverse pride in my second Tale, as scurrilous as it will seem. I don't ask for forgiveness or even understanding, but merely that you read it. It appears here only because it is my price for telling the ductus story, and perhaps my confessional after all these years.

Unlike most of the residents in training of those days, I was a married man, having had a formal military wedding during the war. The ceremony took place just before I was to go overseas, and, as in so many of the weddings performed under such circumstances, had an air of urgency about it because none of us in uniform had any idea whether we would be coming back. And also as in so many of the weddings performed under such circumstances, my wife and I realized when the war was over that we were mismatched. We tried to make a go of it for the first few months, but to no avail. I don't know how my wife handled the situation (and it may say something about me that I didn't care), but as for me, I began having brief flings with student nurses, who thought of me as some sort of desirable war hero, which I certainly was not.

Canterbury Hospital was a much smaller place in those days, and most of the staff, professional and otherwise, were familiar with one another. Accordingly, it was necessary to be very discreet about illicit couplings, and to seek out hiding places and times at which discovery was least likely. My favorite location for quick assignations was the area adjoining the OR, where a new surgical pavilion was being built, secure particularly because it was festooned with a large sign that read: NO ENTRY UNDER ANY CIRCUMSTANCES—THIS MEANS YOU! The sign was necessary because a large part of the space was still in such unformed condition, and entering it was very hazardous.

But late-night prowlings had made the location very familiar to me, and I knew a particular spot where the workers had placed an old and somewhat tattered sofa on which several of them customarily ate lunch each day. About once a week, always during the midnight-to-8:00 A.M. shift, I would lead some attractive young thing to the very place, and cohabit with all the hurry demanded by such conditions.

The Tale of this particular piece of tail took place about six weeks before my adventure with the ductus. I had developed a reputation around the hospital as a very skillful surgeon and a clever diagnostician, as well as being virtually the right-hand man of the great and all-powerful Professor Carl Swenson. It didn't hurt that the fiction of my having been some sort of war hero was well known. To members of the hospital administration, I could do no wrong.

But I was no hero to Hilda McIntire, the maiden-lady night nursing supervisor, who seemed, for whatever reason, to harbor some dark suspicion about the way I used my eminence to get special favors from various levels of personnel. I had always guessed that she knew of the unhappy state of my marriage and the solution I had found for it. Several times during my nocturnal wanderings, I had even wondered whether she was tiptoeing a corridor or two behind me, just to be sure that I was really making night-time rounds and not merely looking for an available conquest.

On the night of this Tale, I was on the couch for a quick tryst with one of the probationers, as they were then called, when a large, gleaming flashlight suddenly illuminated the entire area with a beam as bright as any I had ever seen on a battlefield or aid station. There was Hilda McIntire, having caught her prey at last. And there was I, with my fly open and my probie's underpants lying not far away on the floor.

McIntire made no secret of her intentions, nor of her unalloyed pleasure at finally having trapped her quarry. "What a disgrace you are to this great institution, Dr. Catledge— shame, shame, shame! I'll see to it that you're out of here by tomorrow—and that goes for you, too, Miss Krajewski!" And with that she left as fast as her virginal legs would carry her.

But my arresting officer had forgotten to take one consideration into account: She was dealing with a man who had spent three years in the army as a medical officer, and who was familiar with every form of subterfuge of authority known to such as me. No sooner had the sound of her heavily starched uniform become inaudible than I decided upon my plan of action. Assuring my young companion that she had nothing to worry about, I gingerly escorted her back along the planks and railings of the construction site and went off to practice my newly invented story on an intern I chanced to come across, still awake because he had just admitted an injured drunk from the emergency room.

My plan was to get to Dr. Littlefield, the executive president of the hospital, before McIntire did, which was not much of a challenge because she had to deliver her morning report to the day-shift supervisor before she could do anything else. No sooner had Littlefield unlocked the door to his office at 7:30 A.M. than I stepped in behind him, my face flushed (I have no idea how I faked it) with self-righteous anger. "You won't believe this," I said, barely able to choke back my phony wrath, "but I caught Miss McIntire in the restricted construction area about four o'clock this morning. I have no idea what she was doing there, but this is not the first time I've wondered why she sometimes can't be found for a half hour at a time during her shift." Of course, I had no basis for such an accusation, but how was Littlefield to know? "Do you suppose she sneaks off to have a nip at a bottle of Scotch or something?"

The war hero with an impeccable reputation had just accused the night nursing supervisor of being a drinker or, worse yet, a full-fledged alcoholic who secretively entered an expressly forbidden area of the hospital to do her tippling. Oliver Wendell Littlefield, upright Yankee that he was, needed not a word of further testimony. He was jury and judge, and would do the right thing by the reputation of Canterbury Hospital. He asked me to stay until Hilda McIntire arrived after turning over her shift. When she appeared half an hour later to make her accusation, he was ready for her. He would not hear a word of what he considered to be an implausible story made up to cover her indiscretion. He fired her on the spot and thanked me for saving Canterbury from any further damage Miss McIntire might have done, had she ever made some dreadful and irretrievable error while in an inebriated state.

❧

Commentary to
The Chest Surgeon's Tale(s)

He's right, of course: Henry Catledge was a scoundrel. The reasons are obvious and hardly need rehearsing, but there were others as well. To begin with, he had no business being in the operating room watching that ductus being done: He was supposed to be in Room #4 assisting an intern remove a benign tumor from the skin of the chest wall. But he had left that to one of his assistants because he found the ductus more interesting, which some might consider a dereliction of duty, especially because the assistant was not particularly experienced and the intern had never operated before. Swenson was noted for not looking up when he dissected, being one of those totally focused surgeons who keeps his gaze fixed on the sterile field, so he'd failed to notice Catledge's great skinny length coming closer and lower just before that final ridiculous moment.

But that was only one of the younger man's sins. Catledge could never keep his mouth shut, and it was hardly a secret that he'd been having momentary affairs with student nurses, though no one knew where he carried them out. The word had gotten to Swenson as a bit of a rumor, but he already had strong suspicions that the rumor was based on truth. In his own indirect way, in fact, he'd spoken to Catledge about what he'd heard, and warned him that this kind of behavior, if verified, was not going to be tolerated. Though he never could prove a thing about the firing of Hilda McIntire, he had his own thoughts about the matter.

And then there was Catledge's well-known habit of stealing cases from junior residents. As much surgery as he had done in the army, he was always looking for more. So if there was an operation that a third-year resident, for example, might just about be ready for, the enthusiastic young man could show up in the OR only to be told by one of the nurses that his senior had decided to do it himself. Or should Catledge actually do the assisting, he tended to be so impatient that the junior was often hurried along at a pace for which he was not yet sufficiently skillful, which sometimes led to dangerous circumstances that might have been avoided with just a bit of patience.

And of course, Catledge was no war hero. Though he tries in the telling of his Tale to sound more modest than he was, the fact is that he was prone to drop hints to impressionable medical interns and nurses that his exploits in the military were far more extensive than they had actually been. The result was that more than a few of the younger people on staff had the impression that he had frequently asked for especially hazardous duty or risked his life to save a comrade. The truth, as we knew from Jerry Marsden, who had served with him as a superior officer, was that Henry was constantly trying to be assigned to rearward stations, and only a few times gotten—always unavoidably—anywhere near real action.

And then there was the matter of his marriage. Mary Haines was the daughter of a wealthy Boston family, and her romance with the dashing captain whom she married just before he shipped out to Europe had been the kind of whirlwind in which many young people were becoming involved at that time. Had anyone in her family made more than the most superficial of inquiries, they'd have discovered that he had used every maneuver short of desertion to avoid overseas duty, including a few that made the McIntire caper seem tame by comparison. He had presented himself to the Haines family as being one of three brothers, the other two of whom were decorated pilots—the truth being that one was a civilian motorcycle mechanic and the other a supply sergeant permanently stationed near home at Fort Dix. These are relatively small lies and would have been unnecessary but for Catledge's need to present himself as something he was not. It certainly would have made not a whit of difference to Mary had she known she was marrying the son of a New Jersey truck farmer, but he nevertheless found it necessary to describe his father as the district attorney of a small county in Pennsylvania. More an elopement than the formal military wedding Catledge describes, the hurried affair was attended by no one from his family. Within weeks of her new husband's leaving for Europe, Mary Catledge knew the whole truth. Though not the sort of woman to be disappointed by the facts, she was devastated by the dissimulation. Actually, a good example of that dissimulation is to be found in his Tale: "My wife and I realized when the war was over that we were mismatched." Though they were indeed mismatched, the real problem was that Mary had been deceived. There was a bit of the sociopath about Henry, and Mary was well rid of him. Ironically, she would in later years marry the district attorney of a small town in Pennsylvania.

These kinds of stories, characteristic of Catledge's perfidy, had filtered their way among enough of the medical staff that nothing he did in his later career ever surprised anyone. You will recall that he describes himself as twenty years later being "a professor myself at a reasonably good university hospital." The story of his ascension to that post is vintage Henry. Having completed his training in Michigan, he was appointed instructor in chest surgery at a new medical school that might with some charity be called third rate, located in a small industrial Midwestern city. Whatever else might be said of Henry Catledge, no one who knew him could possibly deny that he was a gifted surgeon and a skilled diagnostician, as he correctly describes himself. But those qualities alone are not sufficient to carry a man to the level of full professor, especially in a school attempting to improve its virtually nonexistent reputation in academic medicine. As always, however, Henry had a scheme. Shortly after arriving at the new institution, he began romancing the spinster daughter of the town's biggest steel magnate. But this time he was in no hurry: The person really being romanced was not Harriet Buchdrucker, but her father, Oscar, who was not only the president of the steel company, but also a director of the area's leading bank, though not very sophisticated in the ways of universities.

Harriet was flattered by Henry's attentions, but Oscar even more so. He did everything he could to encourage the slowly budding romance between his daughter and the desirable young surgeon, but Catledge continued to move slowly. Despite that lengthy scarecrow physique, he was a handsome man, and as charming as such schemers so often are. He kept Harriet on a long string while dating some of the town's more attractive young women, a few of whom were war widows who fell for the hero image as though they had found the reincarnation of an idealized husband no longer alive. Of course, in that faraway place, nothing of Catledge's reputation ever surfaced, and he played the part of rising young surgeon as though auditioning for a movie. Somehow, the story got around of a first marriage, but Henry played it as tragedy, with a beautiful young wife taken early by a rare blood disease.

Henry had more than a thin streak of envy in him. He was bothered by the fact that so many of the men with whom he had trained before the war and at Canterbury were rising in the academic ranks, and he was determined to do the same. He wanted nothing so much as the title of full professor, and the distinction of being elected to several of the elite surgical societies. It was by romancing Harriet, and through Harriet romancing Oscar, that the—here's that word again—scoundrel saw his way. Bit by bit, he stopped dating the belles of the town and began concentrating so much on Harriet that Oscar was becoming increasingly convinced that his plain-faced, ungainly daughter might yet win the big prize. As though baiting a hook, he donated $50,000 to the medical school's department of surgery and was put on the hospital board. The next step, which took place two years later, could have been predicted by anyone who knew Henry Catledge— now thirty-eight years old and just becoming silvery gray at the temples—from his salad days: An engagement of marriage was announced between Miss Harriet Schaufenster Buchdrucker and Dr. Henry van Cleve Catledge III, with the wedding to take place at a date some eight months hence. When the news reached Canterbury, no one was surprised at the van Cleve (which was legitimate and had been very helpful in Henry's youthful and later roamings), but the III was greeted with the amused surprise—well, maybe less surprise than might be thought, considering the other imaginary parts of his history—that it merited.

If any marriage ever deserved the designation "of convenience," the match bringing together Harriet Buchdrucker and Henry Catledge (and, not incidentally, Oscar) was the one. In its honor, the Oscar Kurt Buchdrucker Chair in Thoracic Surgery was announced, with Henry as its first incumbent. Everybody won: Harriet got the most desirable catch in town; Henry got his endowed chair and the national recognition that came with it; and Oscar, the biggest winner of all, married off his quite ordinary daughter to a professor of surgery and had his name memorialized for all time, the whole package at a cost of perhaps $2,000,000.

Over the years, Henry had made so much of his (foreshortened, but few remembered that, or cared anymore) period of training with Carl Swenson that the president of the American College of Surgeons chose him to introduce the honoree on the evening of his retirement. And so it came to be that Henry Catledge achieved what few would have believed possible on that day two decades earlier when he ran clumping and thumping out of OR #3 with the infuriated Carl Swenson hot on his pail-impaled trail. He had, as the more than slightly inebriated Swenson pointed out at that moment, "recovered as well."

I dare Henry Catledge to deny a word of this story.

꘎

The Medical Student's Tale

T HOUGH THIS STORY TOOK place when I was a medical student, the Narrator has very kindly consented to
let me include it in his book. Despite all subsequent
experiences, it remains the most fascinating case I have ever
seen. So what does it matter if it happened before I officially
had my M.D.?

The Tale begins at about 11:00 on a Saturday evening in the
Canterbury emergency room, where I was on my first rotation
at the beginning of the third year, in mid-June. Interestingly,
the Narrator, though some four years younger than I, was my

supervising intern, a situation not as strange as it sounds looking back on it. I had been a newspaper reporter, was drafted into the Korean conflict, then set my sights on medical school, and was now five years behind academically. I was married, had two small children, and considered the sanctity of the family as my main goal in life—I still do, in fact. Chip, as I'll call the then twenty-four-year-old Narrator, still had plenty of growing up to do, and thought of himself as free as a butterfly among the rose gardens of nurses that Canterbury represented in those days. But even he was stunned by what we encountered that night, in the form of a young man called Peaches Pasqualoni, brought into the ER by his distraught and chubby little wife and his mother-in-law, bearing a horribly swollen and tender mound where his genitals should have been. Penis, foreskin, and scrotum were all involved, as was the surrounding epidermis. The skin over the genitals was so tightly swollen that it no longer had that characteristic inflamed look which the ancient Greeks called rubor, being more like a handful of doughy, dripping, and foul-smelling flesh pressing forward from the angle of his thighs. Neither Chip, Ernest Ranny—the chief resident—nor I had ever seen anything like it. For want of a better name we temporarily called it a genital cellulitis, the latter word meaning a general inflammation of the cellular tissue, especially of the fatty tissues beneath the skin. One of its remarkable characteristics was a series of pinpoint holes perforating the foreskin, where the victim's mother-in-law had inserted needles in the hope of draining some of the purulent fluid. Each of these holes was now dripping, but not enough to lessen the tightness of the entire mound.

History? There was no history—at least at first. The bustling mother-in-law had nothing to say except a belligerent unintelligible groan now and then, delivered in the dialect of some obscure southern Italian town, and the young man himself seemed so determined to keep his secret that we knew he'd not divulge any information except under extreme duress. The key seemed to lie with the chunky little wife, who would, whenever the blond, blue-eyed Chip addressed her, smile shyly as though the keeper of a tightly held secret. Quite obviously, she knew something that might be divulged with the right kind of persuasion.

Finally, Mary Vigliotti, the head nurse, whispered something in Chip's ear and he visibly blanched. Mary said a few words to the wife, Lucianna, and it could be told just by watching the transaction that she had given the younger woman permission to talk. They retired to the nurses' station, from which a few minutes later Chip emerged with the spilled beans in his hand. Lucianna stood behind him arms akimbo, smiling at his obvious discomfiture. The story we then heard so infuriated me that Ranny let me lead the surly troop into the cubicle where the young man had been placed, and then to conduct the questioning, very much as follows, as I stood at the foot of the gurney firing one angry question after another at my hapless, suffering patient:

"Your name is Pasquale—otherwise known as Peaches—Pasqualoni and you're married to Lucianna?

"Yeah, doc."

"And last night, with full knowledge of Lucianna and your mother-in-law you went to what they call 'Italian Night' at a whorehouse on Judge Avenue?"

"Yeah, Doc."

"And you and your pals had your cocks sucked like you do every Friday night after supper, right?"

"Yeah, Doc."

"But last night wasn't enough for you and you gave the whore a few extra bucks and stayed about an hour and a half instead of your usual half hour, getting slurped with all that girl's might—tongue, teeth, and all, am I right?

"Yeah, Doc, but you have to understand—"

"That's the trouble, I do understand. What I do understand is that it's been a custom for generations for young, married men from your town and near it to go off together and get blowjobs after dinner on Friday. And every one of the wives not only knows about it, but thinks it's a way for the boys to let off steam so they themselves don't get bothered. Their grandmothers allowed it—even encouraged it—in the old country. It wasn't considered sex, so no marriage vows were broken."

"Yeah, that's right, but what can be done about it? Watcha gonna do to save my cock?"

Here, Ranny could no longer resist. "Listen, kid, what's more important to you, your cock or your life?"

"What kind of question is that to ask, Doc? It ain't that bad, is it?"

"Well, unfortunately it *is* that bad, because the most poisonous animal bite comes from the human, and that broad must have given you a good nip half a dozen times at least. We're taking you up to the operating room, to see how much we can save."

The response was almost a shriek now: "Oh, oh, oh, please don't cut my cock or balls off!"

"We'll do what we have to do in order to save your life, and nothing less."

Appropriately terrified, the boy was taken up to the OR, where Ranny let me make a few longitudinal cuts into the hugely swollen foreskin and then slide a series of slip drains into every possible opening we could find in the tissues. Penicillin, streptomycin, and tetracycline had been started in the emergency room. The final outcome would depend, as it so often does in cases both larger and smaller than this one, on nature's will.

Slashing into Peaches's pus-filled foreskin did not ameliorate my anger, nor lessen the thoughts of my wife and two babies at home. I asked for the responsibility of changing the daily dressings, and Ranny let me take it.

Those were my two favorite times of the day. Morning and evening, I would vengefully march into the four-bed room where Peaches was boarded, and he'd turn white at my appearing there. I'd do it the same way each time: As he strained to look, I'd peel the wet dressings down, look mournfully at the warped, corrugated-looking mess of the boy's genitals, and make the same morose pronouncement: "Too early to tell." (Or, if I felt really sardonic, "Not improving as fast as it could.") I'd then pour a chloride solution called Dakin's on the tissues along with new wet dressings and wordlessly march my pessimistic way out of the ward. Of course, my little game was up on the fifth day, when Ranny came in and took out the catheter, signaling sufficient healing for the boy to pee unassisted. Three days later, the dressings were discontinued entirely and I lost my status as avenging angel. But it was a great ride while it lasted.

Addendum:

In later years, Peaches became prosperous as the owner of a string of three dry-cleaning establishments in our small city. When he was elected Alderman Pasqualoni, one of his first official acts was to publicly close down the whorehouse where Italian Night was held every Friday. He and his svelte blond wife, Lu (née Lucianna), were soon pillars of the community.

The Geriatrician's Tale(s)

I SOMETIMES THINK OF GERIATRICS as the oldest and yet the newest form of medicine. It is a specialty whose full value was recognized only a generation ago, and yet, in a sense, it has been with us forever. Nursing homes for the elderly and infirm have been a constant presence since the Middle Ages, but the technologically equipped, highly trained geriatrician of today is a relatively modern phenomenon, especially when he or she crosses specialty boundaries to work in coordination with, for example, an orthopedist or a cardiologist. It is not hyperbole to claim that a geriatrician is the family physician for the elderly, just as the pediatrician serves that function for the youngest of our population.

Sensing a need in our Canterbury Department of Medicine, I chose to study geriatrics long before it was associated with prestige, government grants, and the sophisticated research of today. I was, in a way of speaking, in on the ground floor, so I have many stories to tell. I've chosen two, not so much for their being remarkable, but because they represent the wide variety of patients who cross the thresholds of our offices and clinics.

All doctors have stories to tell about the cards, letters, or gifts they receive each anniversary of an operation or other successful treatment, or perhaps on Christmas or another holiday, to thank them once again for the care received—and sometimes the life saved—years before. I'm no different from anyone else in this regard, but I do have a favorite among them. For the past twenty years, I've been the recipient of cards on every conceivable holiday from one particular woman whose case history epitomizes to me the way today's super-technology blends effortlessly with the principles of physical examination put forth by the Hippocratic physicians of 2,500 years ago. But it's the physical examination I'd like to describe first, in fact the part of it that may be the easiest though most overlooked: simple observation.

Jean Michaels had been suffering from painful ankle joints for almost a year when she was referred to me by her family physician from a town about twenty miles away. At fifty-eight, she was below the age range of my usual patients, but her doctor assumed, and correctly so, that geriatricians are more likely to be interested in nontraumatic painful joints than would an orthopedist. There was, he told me, a significant discrepancy between the degree of pain and the objective findings in his patient's ankles, including an only slightly abnormal X-ray. Numerous treatments had been tried to no effect, and he was now reaching out in the hope of providing this emotionally stable woman some relief. There was nothing in her history or life situation that made him suspect that he might be dealing with psychosomatic pain, and he had become convinced that he was missing something.

He proved to be right. As I was carefully examining each of her other joints for some clue, I was struck by a phenomenon called clubbing that she exhibited in her fingertips. Clubbing is the name given to a deformity that creates the appearance of a rounding of the connection of the nail bed near its attachment to the finger, so that the entire fingertip looks a bit like a flattened club or spoon. No one really knows how it comes to be, though it is commonly found in children whose blood is not carrying enough oxygen, as often happens in congenital heart disease. But it is also seen in occasional cases of lung cancer, and here, too, no one precisely understands why this should be. When I pointed out the clubbing to Mrs. Michaels, she was impressed by the changes in her fingers, which had apparently occurred so subtly over the past year that neither she nor her doctor had taken notice of them. When a chest film that afternoon showed a vaguely suspicious area in the upper portion of her right lung, the radiologist went on and did a computerized tomography scan of the area, which showed a small cancer. This would also explain arthritis symptoms out of proportion to the actual findings.

I sent Mrs. Michaels to see Sam Carstairs, who was at that time about to succeed Carl Swenson. It was his difficult job to tell her that lung cancers, no matter how small, have a particularly poor prognosis when they are accompanied by peripheral symptoms like clubbing and arthritis, which have no physical relationship to the tumor itself. She accepted the news stoically, told her family, and arranged for the surgery. To the surprise of everyone but Carstairs—who had seen this outcome several times in the past—our patient woke from the anesthesia without any of her previous arthritis pain. Over the course of the next six months, her clubbing disappeared as well. Throughout careful and frequent follow-up, she has never demonstrated any recurrence of her lung cancer in all of these twenty years. And that explains why I get one of those cards on every occasion that provides an excuse for it. Carstairs gets one at Christmas, and the original referring doctor—well, he gets none at all.

MY SECOND TALE IS OF quite a different sort, one in which a discarded and dangerous medication is rediscovered as a useful and safe one for a disease that has defied medical efforts for generations. And best of all, it is rediscovered by a man who had suffered from the disease for decades, despite the best of medical help. No one, including Hulusi Behcet, the Turkish dermatologist who initially described and characterized the disease during the first part of the twentieth century, has had any idea of its cause, though there have been plenty of notions about how to treat it, ranging from cortisone preparations to anticancer drugs (Behcet's disease, as it is called, is not a cancer) to steroids. However, none of these has been universally satisfactory, and each seems to be restricted in use to specific manifestations of the illness.

The most prominent evidence described by Behcet is a prevalence of ulcers in and around the mouth as high as 97 percent, with 83 percent of patients being plagued by genital ulcers and 75 percent having skin ulcers elsewhere. About half of patients also have uveitis, inflammation of the tissue of the eye. Fortunately, the disease is not common, for the suffering caused by it is formidable—physically and esthetically.

Franklin was referred to me when he was in his sixties, having had the entire spectrum of treatments for various of the disease's unbearable burdens, including multiple eye operations that had left him with monocular vision. Fortunately the disease is not hereditary, but it does seem to have clusters in individual families. For such reasons, many patients with early Behcet's never consider marriage, even were they to find a lover who was not put off by the appearance of a potential mate with ulcers of the mouth and genitals.

Franklin had been treated with chronic cortisone therapy and had for a long time been taking the anti-immune medication cyclosporine, but these had barely kept his problems in check. Unlike many patients, he had not pursued the leads offered by alternative medicine, because none of his friends had ever benefited by any of the various recommended nostra.

Franklin had developed a regularity of life that seemed to suit him, though I'm sure he'd have preferred to be more involved with the outside world. Working at an office job as a patent attorney's assistant suited him fine, but a social life built around living with his two spinster non-Behcet's sisters did not suit him at all. As he came closer to retirement, his vistas widened, and he began to seek treatment by any manner that held promise so long as they weren't folk or naturopathic. He had recently discovered the Internet, but everything he came up with was, as he called it, more of the same, with nothing new appearing to have any interest for him.

And then one day he surprised me by coming into the office with a suggestion that he'd found on a Behcet's website, touting the effects of thalidomide for his condition. He asked to try it because it was something with which he'd had no experience, and I promised to do what I could. "Yes, yes, Doc," he assured me. "I'm well aware of the horrible congenital deformities in the babies born of mothers in the 1960s who had used thalidomide as a sedative, and I know that the stuff has been long off the market, but can we just get some and try? After all, I'm not pregnant, you know."

I did my homework, and to my amazement found some very early studies indicating that this medicine might indeed be helpful, but it had been discarded for all uses after the tragedies of the early 1960s. The drug not being FDA approved, it took Franklin and me about six months to push it through our Human Investigations Committee and the Food and Drug Administration's complex paperwork to get proper sanction.

And then the excitement began. Several weeks after starting on the new therapy, Franklin's ulcers began to heal, and before much longer I was able to get him off the dreaded steroids with their frequent complications. I tried the stuff on a few other patients and they all improved, though his success was the greatest. Ten years later, Franklin is doing well off steroids or any other medications, and several studies from other centers have confirmed the potential effectiveness of the drug in a number of small groups of patients.

☙

Commentary to The Geriatrician's Tale(s)

I would claim that the diagnostic and therapeutic epicenter of a modern hospital is its emergency room. It is the place from which everything else seems to radiate. And it is at the same time the hospital's show window—the area that demonstrates not only to the local citizenry and perhaps the world what can be done in the institution, but to its staff as well. Nowadays, it functions as the hub of the scientific practice of the most advanced forms of medicine.

Which is why it seems ironic that, midway through writing this past chapter, I found myself a patient in one of the busiest and most highly regarded emergency rooms in the northeastern part of the United States. I was ambulanced there because of a combination of abdominal pain and a state of dehydration so severe that I could not walk without staggering, or climb stairs without clutching the banister. As in most emergency rooms, I had plenty of time to muse, and the major object of my thoughts was the marked difference between this facility and the calm, unhurried way in which geriatricians go about their daily doings. In the geriatrician's hands, the high tech comes only after the careful evaluation of a history and physical exam. In the emergency room philosophy, things are quite different.

My care in the ER was seen to by a medical student and a doctor in residency training, though it is only fair to say that an attending emergency physician spoke to me several times over the raised bars of my gurney. These three attractive young people could not have been kinder, gentler—as were the very capable nurses—nor more considerate of my moment-to-moment personal needs. What astonished me was their handling of my *medical* needs. In spite of hearing from a seventy-seven-year-old man that he'd been staggering, no attempt was made at a neurological exam. The abdominal evaluation consisted of a few diffident palpations of my lower quadrants and no rectal examination despite a history of treated prostatic cancer. The CT scan was the determining factor in deciding that I had no serious intra-abdominal pathology. All (including my lab tests) agreed that I was quite dehydrated, and I was infused with two liters of saline before being allowed on my way.

I cannot help but contrast all of this with the image of Liam Curray carefully inspecting the fingernails of a woman whose complaint was ankle pain, and as a result coming up with a life-saving diagnosis of treatable lung cancer. I say this not so much to fault the young doctors, because this is the way they are being trained to function in a busy emergency room. But the fact is that they evaluate patients very much in this way in the in-patient divisions as well, where there is much more time to act and to think, and plenty of senior faculty to consult. I am adding nothing but yet another personal experience to the many such stories told of the mechanization of medicine, but I do have one contribution to make and it has to do with geriatricians. Geriatricians treat each patient like a fine old engraving, any line of which may have significance that would be overlooked were it not observed so meticulously. They carefully select more technological diagnostic options only after knowing of such matters as social circumstances, patterns of living, and daily activities. Therapy is directed at an entire way of life, rather than merely the acute problem that brought patient to doctor. This is one-on-one medicine, and the younger geriatricians have been taught it in the same way by their seniors.

Doctors are inordinately fond of saying that their best teachers are their patients, but this is true only when each patient is allowed to teach. A hurried examination and history-taking is not a teaching session, and neither is a routinized therapy.

Much of this kind of teaching by careful study of patients actually goes on during the physical exam, and present-day doctors are cheating not only the sick but themselves by short-shrifting it. This has been well known since approximately 300 BCE, when careful inspection and palpation were introduced by the physicians of the Hippocratic era. In addition to noting the quality and rate of the pulse, such findings as skin turgor and color, characteristics of hair and its distribution, appearance of the tongue and oral membranes, and similar matters were recorded, as were the size of the liver and spleen.

Except for minor modifications, the physical examination remained essentially unchanged until it was pointed out by the Italian anatomist Giovanni Morgagni, in the mid-eighteenth century, that patients' symptoms could be correlated with findings discovered at autopsy after their death. In the new spirit of inquiry that arose after the revolution of 1789, French physicians used that discovery to develop a method of predicting the autopsy findings by systematic physical examination of the living patient, similar to the one honored by the profession until the present generation. The high point of this period of development came in 1819, when René Laennec of Paris published a remarkable little book called *On Mediate Auscultation,* in which he reported a variety of sounds that could be heard when a new instrument of his invention, the stethoscope, was interposed (therefore *mediate*) between the ear of the listener and the chest of the patient, a process called auscultation. This new instrument allowed a novel way of discovering pathological changes in the underlying lung, and heart as well, while the patient was still alive. The quartet of techniques called observation, palpation, percussion (tapping), and auscultation became the hallmarks of the physical examination, and so they have remained until recently. Each of them is obviously applicable to areas of the body other than the chest.

The physical examination is not only a method for diagnosis, but serves in more subtle ways as well. Most specifically, it is a means of contact between doctor and patient. The laying on of hands, as it were, allows two human beings to touch each other in an unthreatening mutual transmission of discovery. A relationship is changed by it, often to one of more intimacy and trust. When it is hurried and perfunctory, one type of message is conveyed; when it is warm and caring, quite another. Either way, each participant learns something about the other and is likely to feel emotionally closer thereafter. If nothing else, it sends a note of caring from doctor to patient.

And, of course, a great deal can be learned from a carefully conducted physical examination. Such findings as appearance, tenderness, texture, organ size and shape, spasm, and auscultatory disclosures may not only lead to diagnosis but often give a clue as to which other, more complex, tests are appropriate, rather than relying on the wide, scattershot guessing so prevalent today. It has been remarkable to me to note how many of the positive findings on the typical abdominal computerized tomography scan can be picked up by wise examination of the abdomen, especially when combined with a simple X-ray film of the area. This is often true of the chest as well. I do not advocate trying to save money by avoiding necessary scans and similar studies, but there is no question that medical costs mount when physical examination is ignored or downgraded. A careful history-taking and physical examination will accurately diagnose appendicitis approximately 90 percent of the time, and yet it is unusual nowadays for a CT scan to be missing from the workup of a patient with appendicitis symptoms.

This, of course, is one of the reasons for which I admire geriatricians so much. Not only are such factors as the social history so important to their completed evaluation, but the unhurried physical examination is essential. I have never watched a geriatrician work without making note of his or her meticulous attention to such matters.

The Bronchoscopists's Tale

M Y NAME IS BOTU Adunabadajo, but that hardly
makes a difference, because I use it only when I
need an alias. Also, it's the kind of alias a hearer is
apt to forget in a minute, so such a name adds to its own—and
my—anonymity.

The passport name I was using from Lagos to London, on
the other hand, is Reginald Farnsworth, which was given to me
by a well-meaning English visitor when I was three. It had always
been everyone's intention that I be a surgeon, and Reginald with
the added Farnsworth seemed more acceptable to most than a

backwoods name like Botu, which is, in any event, well shared among most of the regional tribes.

In the tiny tribe into which I was born—and in many other regional groups as well—Botu means "one who has had his left middle finger amputated at birth," hardly a quality helpful in the operating theater. Such a mutilation does have its uses in my own community, though, because it always signifies the next, or current, bearer of the headmanship of the small village into which one was born.

The main disadvantage, of course, is that an absent middle finger hardly makes for good surgical technique. In fact, after the index finger and thumb, one is more severely handicapped by the absence of that digit than any other. The result is that few have been able to overcome the defect. Believe me, I have seen many a failed surgeon in my part of Nigeria whose only problem was that he was born the son of a local chieftain.

And so, my choice was to not make the attempt. But I have always been fascinated by the notion of being a surgeon, so what is a tall, skinny young black man to do with such ambitions? I elected to become a bronchoscopist.

A bronchoscope is precisely what its name implies: a long— and in those days of the early 1960s, when my Tale takes place, rigid—steel tube which its operator passes through the patient's mouth, then between the vocal chords and down into the trachea, the main passage carrying air into the lungs. In the upper portion of the chest, the trachea divides into two so-called mainstem bronchi, each of which further divides and then subdivides into smaller bronchi like the branches of a tree, and finally into even smaller twigs called bronchioles until the air finally gets to the alveoli, the tiny air sacs surrounded by capillaries, where oxygen is transmitted directly into the blood to combine with hemoglobin for transport throughout the body.

The point at which the trachea splits into the two main-stem bronchi is called the carina. In Latin, *carina* means "keel of a boat," and the line of division has exactly that shape, as each of the two bronchi goes off—to the right and left lungs, respectively—at a somewhat acute angle. Picture yourself having inserted your bronchoscope through the vocal chords of a supine patient and down into the trachea. Directly in front of you is a keel-shaped structure: the carina. You are looking at it through a hinged lens, which can easily be removed should you wish to pass a thin instrument into the depths of one or another of the main-stem bronchi or its branches. By far the most common instruments would be a biopsy forceps or a swab to take bacterial samples.

In the hands of an expert, the bronchoscope is an instrument of invaluable uses. It enables direct visualization into the depths of one or the other lung, biopsy of suspect tissue, and bacterial sampling. A good bronchoscopist is an important asset to the team of the chest, or thoracic, surgeon, who is often present when the procedure—bronchoscopy—is being done, in order to visualize the pathology he or she will have to deal with at operation.

Nowadays, bronchoscopes are fiber-optic and can be turned and twisted down and around all sorts of corners, irregularities, and abnormalities. Also, most present-day surgeons do the procedure themselves. But in 1960, thoracic surgeons in general were likely to have a favorite bronchoscopist, who would do the procedure and report the results.

There were several notable exceptions to this general rule among the surgeons, and the best of them was Sir Russell Sellers, chief of the Thoracic Unit at Middlehammer Hospital in central London. Sellers was so good (one of his favorite expressions when asked to explain his facility with the instrument was "It's all in the wrists, old chap") that problem bronchoscopies were referred to him from all over Europe and Africa.

Sir Russell had spent the entire blitz of World War II in the basement of Middlehammer, doing one after another cadaver bronchoscopy, and in this way wrote the standard text on the structure of the lung as seen from the inside, *The Anatomy of the Bronchopulmonary Segments;* and now, with passport in hand, I, "Reginald Farnsworth," was on my way to London in July 1960 to spend three months at his side learning all of the tricks my brain (and my wrists) could absorb. I had gone to medical school in Lagos, trained in chest disease at Berlin's Charité Hospital, and become quite skilled at bronchoscopy. After visiting the Charité, Sir Russell had invited me to spend the summer with him as part of a program by which he hoped to train certain African physicians, so they might return home and teach special skills to others.

And so the scene is set: The twenty-nine-year-old son (absent his left middle finger) of a Nigerian community chieftain has just arrived in London to learn the highest art of bronchoscopy at the feet (the hands or wrists, truth be told) of the world's expert.

The Tale you're about to read takes place during my second week on the Thoracic Unit. Word has just gotten around that Sellers is about to do the kind of bronchoscopy for which he is most famous: the removal of a small foreign body from deep within the lung tissue of a five-year-old girl. An ambulance is waiting at Heathrow airport for the private airplane of the governor of Gibraltar, whose daughter took a deep breath at the worst possible moment, during an attempt to inflate a large rubber sea serpent whose metallic cap she had secreted in her cheek for safekeeping. Blowing as hard as her tiny, tanned cheeks would allow, she inadvertently inhaled at the wrong instant, aspirating the cap down through her vocal chords and trachea, from where it was swept into the depths of her left lung.

For anyone but Sir Russell, the removal of a distant, deeply buried foreign object from the lung of a small child would represent a formidable difficulty. But this was the man's forte, and he let us know that he would show as many of us as could crowd into his theater just how to do it. His special trainee, "Reginald," would, of course, be at his side.

I overheard the conversation outside the theater as Sir Russell (all five feet eight inches and 150 pounds of him) looked up at Lord Heath (a huge, blustering, florid-faced Colonel Blimp type if ever one such existed) and assured him that he had nothing to fear. Once the anesthesia had been induced, he said soothingly, the actual procedure would take no more than ten minutes, as the cap was found, grasped delicately with biopsy forceps, and brought up into the bronchoscope. The chief made it all sound very easy, though we on his team knew it was a challenging feat—or at least it was a challenging feat for anyone but him.

Excited with anticipation—I perhaps more than anyone else, because these were the kinds of things I had come here to see—our team assembled in Sir Russell's theater, as the anesthetic for this beautiful little blond, blue-eyed girl was quickly and smoothly induced. I stood at Sir Russell's side so that he could talk me through the maneuvers he was using. I had not previously seen a bronchoscope so small as was to be used on the child, and I was more than a little intimidated by its narrow caliber.

The chief advanced the scope deeper and deeper into the tissue of the left lung, and would periodically stop so that I might observe his progress. And then suddenly, there it was: the shiny top of the cap, imbedded in the wall of a very small bronchial branch. With exquisite delicacy, Sir Russell slid the pediatric biopsy forceps down the scope until he could just hear the tap of metal on metal. He stopped again to let several of us see the point of contact, because from here on everything would be done blindly. He twisted his slim wrist delicately, then reported that the cap was now sufficiently loosened from the bronchial wall. I felt sure that the collective sigh of relief could be heard as far away as Gibraltar, as he slowly began to withdraw the forceps with that cap firmly caught in its teeth. When he had the entire apparatus up into the bronchoscope he paused again to let me and his second in command, Harold Ross, see it again. It was a glorious sight: Scope, forceps, and the troublesome cap were in the trachea now, all ready to be lifted out of the child's mouth. As I watched the forceps being pulled upward, Sir Russell, for no explicable reason, must have relaxed the tightness of his grip, and the cap fell loose, clanged down the scope, and bounced off the carina into the opposite side. The foreign body that had been deep in the left lung was now deep in the right lung.

The chief was the only person in the room not horrified. "Well, chappies," he said cheerfully, "here's my chance to demonstrate the procedure again. Rather like a double feature at the cinema, yes?"

The scope was repositioned, and down went the biopsy forceps into the depths of the right lung—once, twice, again and again—each time fruitlessly. The cap could not be located. An X-ray plate was slid under the child and a film taken, but to no avail; it helped not a bit, because it showed only two dimensions. The most self-assured surgeon at Middlehammer had begun to sweat—this was not ordinary perspiration, it was thick, cloying, real sweat, and I could smell it as well as see it come through the armpits of his gown. The theater sister wiped his brow over and over, but nothing could keep it dry. He handed the apparatus to Harold Ross, who made a few passes, but the results were no better.

After almost an hour of trying, the chief had to face the inevitable: To remove the cap, it would be necessary to do a formal thoracotomy, to open little Lucretia's right chest, feel blindly for the foreign body, and then cut through lung tissue to remove it.

The child was turned so that her right side was uppermost, and what seemed like a pint of Merthiolate was swabbed over most of her little body. Sir Russell opened her chest through as small an incision as possible and began to pinch the lung tissue between his long, spidery-thin fingers, in a blind attempt to locate the foreign body where it appeared to be on the radiographic plate. It could not be found.

The chest incision had to be enlarged enough to accept an adult man's hand, which meant the removal of a rib. Only in this way was it possible to locate the elusive quarry. Even after that, it took fifteen minutes of additional dissection to remove it with minimal damage to the lung tissue. This meant that the chest would have to be closed over a tube to contain any air leak.

When the cap was in his hand, Sir Russell flung it to the floor in a gesture of anger or self-contempt, or who knows what? He grabbed me by my bony shoulders and pinned me to the wall as though he were doing it to himself, and shouted, "Now, Botu [Reginald was far from his thoughts at that instant], you've seen how NOT to do it! Perhaps now, dammall, we'll each of us remember that an operation is not over until the operation is over!" He let me go, motioned toward Ross to close the chest, and strode through the swinging doors of the theater, on his way to attempt some explanation to the formidable Lord Geoffrey Heath, the governor of Gibraltar. How indeed had it come to pass that his little girl's right chest was swathed in a large, bulky dressing from which a rubber tube extruded, when she had been flown to London specifically so that the famed Sir Russell Sellers himself should remove a small foreign body from her left lung?

꿍

The Internist's Tale

THE CONTRIBUTIONS—AND ERRORS AS well—of Galen,
the great savant of second-century CE medicine, domi-
nated the art of healing from the time of his career's
height until well into the 1600s, and in certain ways longer. Even
today, there are traces of Galenic terminology in our everyday
speech (when we refer to someone as being sanguine, choleric,
bilious, or melancholic, for example, it is Galen whose words we
are using), and bits of it are still to be found in the clinical jargon
of physicians, who may have no idea of the origins of the terms
tripping so lightly off their tongues.

Somewhere in one of the twenty-two thick volumes left for posterity by the great innovator of Roman times, Galen declared a truth so striking that, should one chance upon it by accident, it is never to be forgotten. In fact, as deeply tucked away in his works as it is, the brief sentence appears to have been known through the ages by more physicians than might be expected from its obscure location: "He cures most successfully in whom the people have the most confidence."

The survival and frequent quoting of this particular truth depend far less, however, on its promulgator's way with words— other writers, before and since, have said much the same thing—than on his reputation as a thoroughgoing pragmatist for whom the rudiments of what then passed for science were paramount, and certainly far more important than the relationship between doctor and patient. That such an unsentimental thinker would pause to consider feelings of this sort must have been startling at the time, and, considering the exalted source, of great significance. That significance has never lessened, though many today who wear the white coat would deny it.

Of course, the fact nowadays is that "he who cures most successfully" is he who most consistently and effectively knows how and when to apply appropriate diagnostic technology of the highest order, obtains the finest super-specialist consultations, and treats with methodologies commonly demanding ultramodern instrumentation. The future promises even more of the same.

But in Galen's day, scientific knowledge was a toddler, barely able to recognize real disease when encountering it. And even as late as the mid-twentieth century, the oncoming flood of the new biomedicine could be described as only beginning to fulfill its potential, though it had traveled a long way toward its present wonderments and was coming closer with each passing decade. Through all of this time, physicians have had ample opportunity to echo—and make use of—Galen's immutable truth. But with the late twentieth and early twenty-first century's outburst of objectified, molecular-based, prospectively double-blinded and meta-analyzed medicine, it would seem that the ancient seer's advice is an interesting—even a quaint—idea, but to many a superannuated one. To plenty of today's physicians, it's nice to be nice, but it's not necessary.

Still, during all of these intervening centuries, most frustratingly including our own, there has always been an occasional patient whose disease has needed more than science can provide, and perhaps even more than the resources of the physician whose command of the molecular basis of healing is greatest. For doctors, the most distressing of these men and women are those whose sicknesses—in spite of modernity's miracles—defy diagnosis and smirk in the face of every therapeutic attempt. They will always be with us.

Some physicians have never had the experience of encountering such a patient; they are the lucky ones. But in the careers of more than a few of us, there have appeared one or two people with such a perplexing array of medical findings that they resist our most wide-ranging experience and ultrasophisticated technologies, not to mention the seemingly endless resources of our great hospitals and the ability to communicate instantly with international authorities. Almost always, such patients will die, sometimes without so much as a diagnosis.

I have been present at several autopsies where even death refuses to yield its secrets to the meticulous probings of which postmortem studies of organs, tissues, and fluids consist; I have seen the most learned of pathologists leave the laboratory as puzzled as their clinician colleagues.

On the rare occasion of being confronted with such a dilemma, I usually find myself developing a particularly close relationship with both patient and family, especially when the clinical course has been prolonged and the frustrations mount with each passing day. Even were one to attempt avoiding such a growing closeness—an avoidance, incidentally, which only a few of us deliberately practice as though it might somehow shield against our own pain—it is virtually impossible. As one diagnostic and therapeutic effort after another is attempted in the hope of solving the insoluble, close bonds inevitably form, whether spoken or simply understood. Elements of deep feeling form a transference to white coat from white sheet, and are returned with a depth of feeling hard for the uninitiated to imagine.

A terrifying and yet somehow mutually supportive comradeship develops in such situations, and it almost invariably includes the family. When it ends in the patient's death, as it almost always does, the tragedy is magnified in its intensity, and has by then come to include nurses, technicians, and ancillary personnel who have also served. It is at such moments that the usual everyday triumphs of medicine lose their meaning, because a friend, the focus of every effort, has died.

And it is also at such moments that Galen's words would seem to have even less significance than usual in our century, for what is the value of all the confidence in the world when there is no cure to be had?

Galen's aphorism is precisely why I have chosen this story as the Tale of my most memorable patient. Harold Bernstein, a forty-five-year-old electronics engineer, was transferred to Canterbury from a small hospital about twenty miles away with the clinical characteristics of a disease called aseptic meningitis, an inflammation of the tissues surrounding the spinal cord, which usually improves on its own with little or no medical intervention. Aseptic meningitis is a nonbacterial process ordinarily caused by a virus, but other organisms may be involved, or even chemical irritants. Its usual presenting symptoms include fever, headache, and stiff neck, all of which Harold had. But when a tap of his spinal fluid on admission made me suspect that this case had additional elements to it, I began to look for some other, less common, cause of his complaints. The looking soon became urgent, because my new patient was clearly becoming sicker by the hour as we observed him, in ways that were consistent with nothing I or anyone on my team had ever seen before.

As the chief of the section of Infectious Disease at Canterbury Hospital, I know a great deal about the wide variety of sicknesses that are caused by organisms originating in the arcane place that Louis Pasteur once called "the world of the infinitely small." The work I do is with bacteria, viruses, protozoa, fungi, and everything else in any way related to a microbe.

My domain extends from strep throat to sporotrichosis, from blastocystis to balantidium, and, importantly for this case, from measles to meningitis. But Harold Bernstein knew within minutes of his spinal tap that I had no idea what was wrong with him. And he knew the day he went home nearly healthy almost five weeks later that I was still no closer to a diagnosis than I had been at that initial hour, or to the reason for his recovery. And he knew something else, too, as did his wife, Etta: Not a single thing that I or my colleagues did had helped him one bit or played an iota of a role in his improvement. He had been cured of some unknown multifaceted and dreadful malady by nature herself. But something within me—something embarrassingly egotistical—likes to think that Galen was right: Harold survived for the simple reason that he was one of those whose doctor can somehow effect a cure when "the people have the most confidence." Or at least that's what Harold says, and I cling to it.

Here is a truism known by every doctor: Now and then it happens that our most grateful patients are those for whom we accomplish the least—sometimes, in fact, those whom we snatch from the jaws of a death in whose vicinity they may not have found themselves in the first place were it not for some well-intentioned but ultimately bone-headed error we had committed. I made no error in Harold's case—at least none I'm aware of—but neither did I do a single thing to help him survive an illness during which he hovered near mortality for more than two weeks, enveloped in a pervasive miasma of ignorance in which I was the central figure.

As we carried out a host of complex physiological and tissue studies, called in one consultant after another, and spent hours reviewing literature and contacting colleagues all over the world, it was becoming increasingly clear that we had no idea where to turn for enlightenment, and our patient was worsening before our eyes. I recall that there was not a single section of the Department of Internal Medicine that we did not call upon for consultation during those first hectic days and thereafter—we even consulted a few surgeons—but no one had anything of value to contribute. By the time we reached the end of Harold's second week in the hospital, he was deeply jaundiced with an unusual form of hepatitis and had severe atypical pneumonia in both lungs, an inflammation of the heart called myocarditis (of unknown cause), anemia, and severe muscle aches, among other debilitating complaints. His recovery seemed unlikely.

Being an engineer married to an architect, Harold, not surprisingly, was accustomed to dealing with very specific information and real data. I would enter his room at least once every day and usually more as his condition worsened, and each time have to tell husband and wife that I was no closer to an all-inclusive diagnosis than I had been when he came through the door. I shared every bit of available information with them and never hid a thing. For reasons I will never fathom, they maintained total trust in what we were doing, even as one after another antibiotic or other pharmacological agent failed to perform as hoped and every diagnostic alley proved blind. Together and separately, both Harold and Etta were told time and again that we didn't really know what we were doing, but each of them somehow managed never to lose that complete trust, even as it was becoming obvious that Harold was closer to death with every passing day of our ineffectiveness. To be told by your patient that he has confidence in you, even as your inability to help him becomes increasingly clear, is to feel like the worst hypocrite in the world.

Within days, we had become like a small family: Harold, Etta, me, and a few of the other doctors trying to help. We shared our fears, our doubts, and our few hopes—but mostly what we shared was our ignorance. Looking back on it, it may have been our complete frankness with one another that maintained the atmosphere of trust. We were flying by the seat of our pants and each of us knew it. Trust, in fact, was all we had to offer one another. "Confidence" was the Bernsteins' word, and they expressed it almost every time we spoke.

Enter Galen—or at least I like to think so. Early in Harold's third week of hospitalization, this very sick man stopped getting worse, for no demonstrable reason. He remained unchanged for a few days, and then one morning I realized that he was the least bit better. Just as his deepening illness had fit no recognizable pattern, his improvement followed no trajectory any of us had ever seen. The one thing of which we were certain was that nothing we had done for him therapeutically could have had any effect. He was doing all of his getting better on his own. He knew it, Etta knew it, and we knew it. Every one of our consultants—personal and electronic—knew it, and no one had an explanation.

The improvement continued. Before two more weeks had passed, Harold was well enough to be discharged home. On subsequent outpatient visits, it was clear that my formerly mortally ill patient was getting better and better, and I still had no idea why. Finally, all that remained of those awful weeks in the hospital was the memory of that plethora of complexities, and the three of us speaking quietly and openly of our thoughts. On each visit, either Harold or Etta or both said what they had always said: They had never lost their confidence in me, misplaced though I knew it to be.

There are those who will read a Tale like this one and invoke all manner of reasons for Harold's recovery, but in order to convince me of any of them they will have to provide a diagnosis as well. This goes for those who prefer the supernatural as well as those others who seek an explanation in something they call psychophysiological (whatever that may mean), and all entries in between.

All doctors—even those who deny it—try to instill confidence in their patients. But only some of us think of it as anything more than a builder of optimism and a source of hope. Some still do consider it an important adjunct to cure. But confidence was all I had to offer Harold Bernstein—there was nothing else. In fact, I'm not at all sure why he did have that confidence. But he had it in good measure, and he is certain that it was the reason for his happy outcome. To this day, five years later, he has had no recurrence.

☙

Commentary to The Internist's Tale

What the internist does not say in his Tale—because his modesty matches his medical brilliance—is that he is the sort of man who could bring confidence to an antelope whose bleeding haunches are being clawed by a hungry lion. Having observed him in the clinics and care divisions of the Canterbury Hospital for so long a time (he is fifteen years my junior), I have been impressed that confidence is an ingredient in every therapy he prescribes for his patients, whether or not he knows it.

Tony Biondi—the Internist—is a small, dark man who is handsome not only in facial features but also in his mien. There is an overt optimism about him, and it cannot but be transmitted to every patient in his care. Though I always tended toward optimism in my clinical work, its opposite is more the attitude with which I face life in general. Were I Tony's patient, I would be an optimist until the day he sent me home recovered.

But though I am writing here about the Tale of a particular physician, I confess that I am to an extent also describing all but the most misanthropic of us. For there is indeed something about the average doctor that inspires at least a degree of confidence, and he or she must do something particularly obnoxious in order to destroy it. An oration delivered by Dr. W. S. Houston at the 1937 meeting of the American College of Physicians was entitled "The Doctor Himself as a Therapeutic Agent," and it dealt with the impact of the healer's authority. In choosing his topic, Houston was following the same line of reasoning as Lewellys Barker, professor of medicine at Johns Hopkins, who had proclaimed in 1908, "Whatever success modern physicians had with their prescribed medications depended largely on their ability to awaken confidence and inspire the idea of authority by their scientific training."

No one knows the effects of thoughts, conscious or unconscious, on the body's response to disease; no one knows the true nature of the placebo effect, for example. Such matters have been studied for decades by an interdisciplinary group representing many distinguished institutions, who have chosen the name psychoneuroimmunology for their field of research, and they report distinct correlations to support their thesis of interrelationships between life events, sickness, and recovery. Many physicians quote anecdotal experience that would seem to support such conclusions, and I have a few of my own, including those that involve the intercession of specific individuals.

But I am here more interested in Tony Biondi himself, and his effect on the undiagnosable and seemingly untreatable Harold Bernstein. For a comment on their relationship—which I believe was one of more than just trust and confidence—I turn to a physician who first wrote about such things half a millennium before Galen. He was either Hippocrates or a contemporary writing in the name of the esteemed Father of Medicine, and this is what he said: "Some patients, though conscious that their condition is perilous, recover their health simply through their contentment with the goodness of the physician."

Regardless of Harold's diagnosis or nondiagnosis, I will always believe that he recovered because of his contentment with the goodness of the physician—not the storied authority of the doctor, concerning which Houston and Barker spoke, and not the trust and confidence to which even the modest Biondi confesses, but that specific quality to which Hippocrates was referring, the simple, unalloyed goodness of a Tony Biondi.

The Surgeon's Second Tale

I BEGAN THIS BOOK WITH a Tale of a young man with a very mysterious condition. The Tale I am about to tell concerns a young man of approximately the same age who also suffered an insult to the diaphragm, but they had very different life experiences.

Jimmy Tyson, as you recall, was a product of the local ghetto, and we never knew a single member of his family, if he had one; Austin Carruthers was a product of Grosse Point, Michigan, and Choate, and was surrounded by a cheerful, loving family of which he was the adored youngest of four children split evenly between boys and girls. Jimmy played no sports, except perhaps street fighting; Austin was an outstanding player on the Canterbury soccer team and a fine amateur boxer. I met Jimmy in a crowded five-bed room on a hospital medical ward; I met Austin in a large, comfortable converted bedroom at the Canterbury Infirmary. Jimmy's chest contained at least a quart of feces-flecked pus; Austin's abdomen was the repository for a fistful of some of the bluest (in the social sense) blood in America.

The Tale of Austin begins at about 5:00 on a lovely spring afternoon in 1965, as I swung by the Canterbury student infirmary on my way from my office in the city. It was my intention to do a postoperative visit on a freshman whose appendix I had removed about five days earlier, and then go back to the hospital for evening rounds. I was about to write a note in his chart describing his good condition when one of the nurses asked me to see a newly arrived sophomore with a self-diagnosed dislocated left shoulder. Feeling inadequate to say much about an orthopedic condition, I tried to demur, reassuring the nurse that one of the bone doctors would no doubt be coming by in less than an hour, and his opinion was worth a lot more than mine. But she was insistent. The boy's pain, she said, was unusually severe for such an injury and she felt that he should not have to wait any longer for a dose of painkiller.

You will understand my reluctance as I stepped into the boy's large corner room. I was surprised to find him sitting bolt upright in bed, his right hand clutching the very top of his left shoulder as tightly as he could. The sitting up, the intense pain, and the tight grasp on the wrong place seemed unusual—that much even I could figure out. I asked him how he knew he had a shoulder dislocation, and between moans he told me that the pain, though much stronger, was reminiscent of what he'd had after sustaining the same injury in high school. But why sit up? "Because," he virtually gasped, "it becomes intolerable when I lie down." When I asked him to describe the mechanism of injury, he remembered only being knocked to the ground and landing on his left rib cage. He had no recollection of his shoulder hitting the ground or being kicked.

Surgeons think of bellies before they think of bones, and my response was immediate. I picked up his bedside phone and called the Canterbury Hospital operating room to tell the head nurse to prepare a room for an emergency splenectomy—removal of the spleen.

The boy's face, which until then had been a normal color, now blanched to a bedsheet white. I sat down at his bedside to convince him that he'd be fine once his bleeding spleen was removed. We had a little talk about anatomy. In what was probably the shortest lecture I've ever given, I explained that the top of the spleen lies in contact with the bottom of the left leaf of the diaphragm, so any inflammation in that region affects both structures. In embryological development, I explained, the nerves (derived from spinal segments 3, 4, and 5 in the neck) to the diaphragm also carry sensation from the top of the shoulder, since they share a common origin in the embryo. Accordingly, when the diaphragm is irritated, the pain often feels as though it comes from the shoulder. "Austin," I explained, "the upper tip of your spleen was cracked when you hit the ground. There's a collection

of blood called a hematoma pushing upward against your diaphragm. The spleen has probably been bleeding slowly, but we
have no idea if or when the drip will speed up."

With the help of one of Austin's roommates, who happened
to arrive for a visit at that time, I took him downstairs and put
him, fully upright, into the backseat of my car with his legs
stretched as far forward as possible. With him in that position,
the spleen would tend to gravitate downward just enough to
provide some relief from the pain.

After a quick stop in the emergency room to record his admission, Austin was taken directly up to the OR. I took advantage of
the time to phone Grosse Pointe and explain the situation to Austin's mother, who gave permission for the surgery. She said that she
and Mr. Carruthers would be at Canterbury within three hours.
When I expressed astonishment at the speed, she told me that her
husband was a senior vice-president at Pan-American Airways,
and a company jet would be made available immediately.

When I opened Austin's abdomen with a generous incision
just below his rib cage, all was as expected. He had a ten-centimeter
leaking hematoma at the top of his ruptured spleen, and it was
pressed tightly up against the diaphragm. Removing the bleeding organ presented no unusual problems, and Austin was in the
recovery room by 8:00 P.M. His parents arrived an hour later.

Austin's postoperative course was smooth, and the little
Pan-Am jet arrived at the local airport seven days later to take
him home for a few weeks' rest before he resumed classes. As I
shook James Carruthers's hand for the last of what had seemed
a hundred times, he thanked me yet again for having saved his

son's life. I am not a modest man, but I told him—as I had before—that training and luck trump brains every time. But he had one last way of thanking me.

"Now remember who I am, doctor. I'm a senior vice-president of Pan-Am, and if there's anything I or my company can ever do for you, just ask."

"Actually," I replied, "I'm taking my wife and two kids to London in August, to visit relatives. Can you help me with that?"

"Say no more, doctor. Just contact me in early July and I'll take care of everything as soon as I hear from you."

Austin was on the plane at that point, so Mr. Carruthers pressed his card into my palm and jumped aboard. He shouted one last "Good-bye and thanks again!" before the hatchway was closed and the plane sped down the runway for takeoff.

I did as I was told. Early in July, I wrote to James Carruthers reminding him of my planned London visit. He was as good as his word; I received a thick envelope from him four days later. I have not seen the accompanying letter in about four decades, but I can quote the second of its two short paragraphs almost verbatim:

"Mr. Carruthers wishes to be remembered to you and thanks you for your services to his son. I have enclosed Pan-Am travel brochures to help you plan your trip. He sincerely hopes you have an enjoyable visit.

Sincerely yours,

Linda Travis

Secretary to Mr. John Carruthers"

The Nephrologist's Tale

T THE AGE OF fifty-five, I'm just old enough to remember most of the rationalizations (and lies) customarily used by admissions committees to deny female applicants a chance to go to medical school. First and foremost, of course, was the old saw that we'd marry before graduating, which would result in the high probability of double jeopardy: "We'll lose not only the woman but also the boy we would have admitted had we not taken her." And then there was the well-worn "We'll accept her and afterwards she'll go on to train in something soft like Pediatrics. Then she'll have her first child and drop out of medicine completely."

And of course, women were thought physically incapable of the long hours of exertion required for completion of a residency training program, and without the manual dexterity displayed by our masculine counterparts. I was told bluntly on several occasions that I seemed to take longer to master some particular technique than did the young man at the adjoining laboratory bench, resulting in much of the instructor's time being wasted. But I always suspected not only that medicine was an old boys' club, but that any boy was thought a great deal smarter than any girl trying to do the same kind of work.

I was never quite sure, for example, whether to be amused or enraged by a statement made in 1850 by the then most outstanding American authority on gynecology, Charles de Lucena Meigs, in a textbook chapter comparing the distinctions that made men more fit than women for certain kinds of undertakings. Referring to gender differences in cranial size, he apparently met no opposition when he wrote, "She has a head almost too small for intellect, but just big enough for love." As a dabbler in medical history, I've never encountered any comment on the meaning of that nonsense, which was a typical reference of the time, pertaining less to the capacity of the cranium than of the intellect. As a medical student in the 1970s, I always suspected being thought less brainy than the gentlemen in my class. That may have been my paranoia alone, but I'm sure that more than a few of the female doctors of the generations before mine would confirm that—at least until the middle of the twentieth century—they were treated almost as though Meigs were still alive and his opinions the gold standard.

But, of all of the accusations made against women as doctors, the one to which I take greatest exception is that we cry too much in the face of our patients' misfortune and tragedy. Of course, my aversion to this particular bit of calumny is very likely because "the lady doth protest too much," since I am certainly one of those profuse weepers. But I have male colleagues far more prone to tears than I am, the big difference between them and me being the effectiveness of my control. Probably because of a hypersensitivity to the charge of emotionalism, I have with superhuman effort taught myself a technique that I refer to as "delayed tearfulness." What I mean by this is that I have somehow learned to hold off until I'm safely in my car before giving in to grief.

Only once in all my years as a kidney doctor (one of those specialties said to be too strenuous for such as me) has any patient or family seen me cry. But that set of circumstances was so unusual that it immediately came to mind when I was asked to describe my most memorable patient.

Lou Rizzo's death made me cry uncontrollably because I had been through one hair-raising medical adventure after another with him during the fifteen years he was my patient; because he had never had the smallest chance of living a life approximating anything like normality; because he was as courageous in the face of the constant chronic threat of dying as anyone I have ever seen; because his demanding personality made him such a pain in the ass that the quality, in time, became endearing; because our most difficult patients are so often those with whom we come to feel the most intimate; and because I had become so close to his mother by the time of Lou's death that I could not help but share her anguish as it burst forth in a single loud wail when she realized that he was no longer alive.

Lou's is a Tale of the sheer burden of disease that one individual may be forced to bear. By the time he died at forty-two he had experienced so much illness, so much diagnostic manipulation, so much surgery of major and minor kinds, and so much emotional trauma that few periods of his life were free of worry or pain. He was born with Type I diabetes of such a serious nature that he developed kidney failure at a very young age and required a transplant from his elder sister when he was seventeen. A few years later, the miracle of a pancreas transplant virtually changed his life—it is no exaggeration to say that he blossomed, and began to feel as though he had at last some chance of being like other young men.

That hope lasted seven years, until the new pancreas began to fail; it could no longer make sufficient hormone to fulfill Lou's metabolic needs. Because the situation had been stable until then, his medical care had been taken over, about two years earlier, by a group of general practitioners. No matter how hard they tried, they were unable to keep him under tight insulin control, and he was once again referred back to our group at Canterbury for attempts at stabilization.

Obviously, a case like Lou's was ideal for teaching, and he was brought one morning to the huge amphitheater where Medical Grand Rounds are held. As always, the first few of the sloping rows were filled with senior faculty, the next few by the middle rank, and the rest in that order all the way back to the medical interns and students high up almost to the ceiling. The occasion was to be used as an opportunity to discuss the advantages and hazards of pancreatic transplantation. The discussants were Josh Davis, chief of the metabolism service, and Vince Fernandes, director of transplantation, who delivered excellent arguments on the two sides of the issue and provided the audience with plenty of information on indications and contraindications.

And then as is customary at Grand Rounds, the patient was brought in. Until that point, Lou had been lying on a gurney in the adjacent hallway, accompanied by a student nurse. Because she was not properly instructed, the young woman had brought his conveyance so close to the entranceway that Lou was able to hear every word spoken, which was not the intent of any of the participants. Though his vision was markedly compromised by the retinal disease—called diabetic retinopathy—that is so often the consequence of many years of the malady, his somewhat surprised facial expression on being wheeled into the auditorium revealed that he had not expected so many to be in the audience. Turning his head slowly from one end of its perimeter to the other, he scanned the entire group as though he were some giant turtle, and then—meekly by Lou Rizzo's usual standards—asked if he could speak.

At such conferences, patients do not ordinarily address the audience except in response to direct questions, so there was a moment's hush of expectancy before Davis hesitatingly assented. And as those who had had any degree of contact with Lou knew, there was good reason for the hesitancy: He was hardly a shrinking violet. He was demanding, opinionated, pushy, loud, and likely to exhibit his own unique brand of angered frustration when refused the thing he had asked for. Given such a large and influential audience, there was no telling to what use he might put the opportunity to speak. Both experts had agreed that another attempt at pancreatic transplant should not be attempted, because of the high failure rate of such operations and the extreme danger to the patient; neither they nor anyone in the amphitheater had any idea that he had been able to hear their decision. Lou had long since become a clinical diabetes expert himself, and there was little except for abstruse biochemical phenomena that he did not understand thoroughly.

Moderately disabled by the long-term neurological effects of his disease—which are collectively called diabetic neuropathy—Lou could not raise himself up on the gurney, but he had no hesitation in asking Davis and Fernandes to help him to a sitting position, with his gnarled, ugly feet hanging over the edge so that everyone could see their twisted, thickened nails and the small skin ulcerations, all caused by the poor pedal circulation characteristic of the chronic diabetic. When the two professors had gotten him propped up this way, one of them took up a post behind each shoulder to be sure their patient was able to maintain balance, as well as to support his back. Of course, he could see neither of them in this position, but it was not Fernandes and Davis to whom Lou intended to direct his remarks. His words were meant for the faculty and students who had assembled in this large academic semicircle to listen to a discussion about the effectiveness of long-term treatment of an anonymous Type I diabetic whose pancreas graft was no longer functioning.

Everyone who spoke up in the prior discussion had agreed that a second attempt at transplant was not indicated; that insulin management would be very difficult; that the patient's history of idiosyncratic and unpredictable compliance with treatment plans aggravated the problems; that there would be many complications and hospitalizations in the coming years. Lou had heard all of it before when he was present at smaller conferences, and never said very much except to utter an occasional grumble of discontent about the medical or nursing care—or the narrowness of the elevators; or the long waits in the X-ray department; or the inedible food; or the roughness of the orderlies; or, or, or, and so forth into a screed of bitching about any of his chronic dissatisfactions.

But in this place at this time, Lou Rizzo suddenly found himself with an opportunity to change some powerful minds. His first few words were spoken with uncustomary softness, as the entire expanse of the audience leaned forward in their seats in order not to miss a single word. As he continued, Lou's voice rose in volume and subtlety of articulation, and yet no listener strained any less, so completely had he captured everyone's determined attention. It was as though a great Shakespearian actor were delivering a soliloquy on what it is like to live one's entire life as a physically and emotionally crippled diabetic.

Lou was describing everyday moments of suffering to which it is impossible to become inured. Though there were certainly at least a dozen diabetics among the faculty and students, no one had experienced even remotely the kinds of anguish that characterized his days, except for the brief seven years when the transplanted pancreas was working with high efficiency. As he made so clear, there was nothing normal in his life, nor the life of his mother, whose almost every waking moment was devoted to maintaining his brittle stability. Everything was aberrant; nothing resembled humanity as it was meant to be.

Though, or perhaps because, I had known Lou for about ten years at this point—knew each bump and bruise in his tragic life—it took every nanogram of my "delayed tearfulness" to maintain some control lest I break down, sitting there in the center of the first row with all the other full professors. Jimmy Eliopolis on my right, Rick Hughes on my left—I didn't have to turn a millimeter to know that they had both begun weeping softly. Barely audible sobs descended from the lofty rows occupied by the junior house staff and students. Lou had not intended for this emotional a reaction; he was not a man who trucked with pathos, for himself or anyone else. His only intention was to let his audience know what it is like to live with his kind of diabetes. But by telling of it with the spontaneity of that distinctive moment was to turn what had been an earnest academic discussion into a candid insight deep within the reality of a life-distorting disease.

Fernandes was trying manfully to stare directly in front of him, but his jaws were twitching tightly, as though to keep his mouth from flying open with a roar of pain at what he was hearing. Davis's way of maintaining control was to stare fixedly at the highest point in the room, just above the head, I suppose, of one of the high-altitude medical interns. By the time Lou asked for a second try at a transplant, Torquemada himself would not have denied him. Lou's retinopathy prevented clear sight of even those of us in the front rows, but he somehow conveyed the impression that he was staring into the eyes of each individual in the entire amphitheater.

Lou's entreaty ended very simply, with exactly the words that were needed: "You have no idea what it's like to be like me. All I want is to be like you." Fernandes and Davis eased him down to a supine posture on the gurney, and the young student nurse—with a faceful of tears and snot dripping onto the collar of her starched blue uniform—wheeled him out of the amphitheater and back to his room.

Though no patient at Canterbury had ever had a second transplant of the pancreas, Fernandes did not hesitate to do one for Lou. But he and his team ignored a single consideration that affected the graft's life far more than surgical skill—namely that Lou was older now, and more noncompliant with his medication program than he had been at an earlier time. When the pancreas was rejected three years later, it was traceable to Lou's having played fast and loose with the immunosuppression drugs. Though he denied it, the evidence was too strong to ignore. He was treated with antilymphocytic globulin, a protein substance that kills the white blood cells called lymphocytes that cause the rejection. The globulin resulted in serum sickness characterized by arthritis and severe general pain, yet another weight added to Lou's increasingly large bundle of difficulties. We did manage to save the pancreas, but supplementary insulin had to be added to the list of medications, and Lou found himself once again in a difficult place.

Meantime, my own academic situation was gradually changing, as I began to be more involved with education and less with the clinical care of patients. Lou's management was turned over to one of the transplant surgeons, who seemed to be somewhat less able to control his medications than others had been in the past, though Lou's contribution to the problem was not inconsiderable. Just about this time, a new transplant director took over, and his first contact with the difficult patient was to see him in the emergency room with chest pain, Lou's diabetes having by now caused coronary artery disease, for which he was being medicated. Because it was obvious that he was acting as carelessly with the heart drugs as he had with so many others, the surgeon read him the riot act, with the result that the offended Lou discharged himself from the ER. A week later, he stormed into the hospital director's office in his wheelchair to complain about how bad his care had been.

All aspects of Lou's disease were now progressing rapidly. The kidney given to him by his sister twenty-five years earlier was failing; he was in chronic congestive heart failure, and was being evaluated for a cardiac transplant; he needed dialysis while plans were being made for the second kidney transplant, but he refused it. In the midst of all of this he sustained a hemorrhagic stroke. Though he was resuscitated, he was left with no brain stem function and transferred to the Neurological Intensive Care Unit, where his mother gave authorization to turn off the respirator the following afternoon.

I went up to the NICU to be with Mrs. Rizzo at the end. Because we had spent so much time together over the years, we were like old friends, and the nurses let us alone with Lou as soon as they disconnected the ventilator. No matter how many times I am present when a respirator is stopped while the electrocardiogram shows a beating heart, I have never gotten used to it. The artificial breathing ends and yet that heart just keeps beating for a minute or more, looking as though it will never quit—until it goes into an irregular rhythm and all is over.

Ida Rizzo did not take her eyes off the electrocardiogram until that microsecond when it stopped and she knew that her son was dead. And then came that single loud wail. I held her close and never stopped to think about this artificial thing I have called "delayed tearfulness." It was time to cry, and I did—with all the unfettered emotion of a woman who has just lost a close friend.

❦

Commentary to The Nephrologist's Tale

It has been about a year since I last looked at the enrollment lists of the senior class at the Canterbury Medical School. The figures were not much different, give or take a few percentage points, than they had been for at least a decade and a half: just about evenly divided, with a slight numerical advantage for the women. When women have dropped out (which they have done in the same percentages as men), it was to spend a year or more doing research in the lab; some have taken maternity leave, but always returned to their profession. In general, the specialties chosen by women seem not to differ in physical or intellectual rigor from those chosen by men. No records are kept about the number of tears shed by one gender as opposed to the other.

It is safe to say that the traditional reasons for refusing women a place in the class have proven to be of no validity, at least for the present generation. The same can be said about relative performance in residency training programs and in the arena of a life in medicine.

There is no way to know if this would have been true a century ago, but one thing is now very clear: Given the same size of applicant pool and the same quality of undergraduate education, men and women will do equally well as medical interns and as physicians. Many observers of the historical scene would be quick to express their opinions that this has probably always been true.

It certainly would have been predicted by the quartet of young women who assembled in 1889 to raise sufficient money to allow the opening of the Johns Hopkins Medical School. That story begins in 1874, when the will of the Baltimore merchant and banker of that name left $7 million of his estate equally divided for the founding of a university and a hospital. The will stipulated that the hospital was to be part of the medical school of the university, by which Hopkins established the precedent that American medical schools are to exist in a university environment of which the teaching hospital is also to be an integral part.

The hospital opened in May 1889, but the inauguration of the medical school had to be delayed because of a large shortage of funds. Mr. Hopkins had invested $1.5 million in B&O Railroad common stock, and new federal regulations had vastly decreased the value of that investment, leaving the new university with a shortfall of half a million dollars. Four young women, all daughters of university trustees, formed a committee promising to raise the money if certain stipulations were met, among them that women be admitted on the same basis as men and that very high qualifications become the standard of acceptance. These were revolutionary concepts that were strongly resisted by the trustees, but to no avail. The money was raised. When the medical school opened in October of 1893, the fifteen men and three women who were its student body fulfilled the most rigorous requirements that had ever been asked of medical students anywhere.

When American medical schools began to pattern themselves after Hopkins in the first third of the twentieth century, they did take on the very high standards, but regrettably had no interest in admitting women on the same basis as men. The result was similar in most institutions to the situation at Canterbury when I was a student there in the middle of the century: a total of seventy-six men and four women. This did not change for another twenty years, but when it did, the change occurred rapidly, for a panoply of reasons. The most important impetus was the women's movement, which gathered force in the 1970s. Once a critical mass of female doctors had entered the workforce, it rapidly became obvious that none of the canards of the past would stand up to reality. And that is why Megan McNally is able to tell her Tale, hidden between the lines of which is the obvious fact that Lou Rizzo had no interest in whether she was male or female. His only interest was in whether he was being treated by the best and most empathic of nephrologists—which he certainly was.

The Neurologist's Tale(s)

WHEN THE NARRATOR APPROACHED me asking for a Tale of the most memorable patient I have ever seen, so many came to mind that making a choice was more difficult than it might, perhaps, have been for most other specialists. No matter how many times I see the same disease, it seems to present itself not only differently, but uniquely, in each patient afflicted with it.

Like the mind, the nervous system is everywhere. Any little manifestation of its possible tics seems to be transmitted to each small area of the thinking and doing parts of us that allow little rest from its manifestations. And those thinking and doing parts respond with messages of their own, so that neurological and mental diseases influence every fiber of what we are, too often in ways about which little can be done. So the patient adapts, and it is in the adaptations that so much of the difference is seen between one person and another.

I have chosen two short Tales to tell, because they lift my spirits and I hope they will lift yours as well. They both involve the kind of tragedy that neurologists face every day, but they both also involve the kinds of adaptation that speak to something in the human spirit that you will recognize, even if few of us can emulate it.

At forty-one, Janice Carpenter, a librarian employed by the city of Los Angeles, had never cared a whit about sports. She never married, as she so often put it, because "I wouldn't know what to talk to them about." All of this became much less of a joke when Janet's health plan physician sent her to consult with me because he was beginning to fear that her slowly increasing muscle weakness might be the harbinger of disease in the motor neurons of her spinal cord, those cells that transmit messages to activate voluntary movement. My workup of her symptoms confirmed his worst suspicions. Janice's diagnosis proved to be amyotrophic lateral sclerosis, called Lou Gehrig's disease for the famous Yankee baseball player whose case first brought the pathology to public notice.

Janice tried to laugh at the irony of this, but she knew too much about the disease to make much of an attempt. In fact, she knew precisely what she was facing over the next three to five years, which is the usual life span of people as the deterioration relentlessly proceeds. But she had the good or bad luck to continue on for at least twice as long as expected, perhaps because of the astonishingly attentive nursing care she was given at a long-term neurological unit within her local university hospital in Southern California. I left for my new post at Canterbury when Janice had been on that unit for a decade, and I later learned that she died the following year.

During my last year at the California hospital I would bring a group of senior medical students to see Janice while they were doing their rotation on our service. The neurology residents had been telling me—and this was confirmed by my own daily observation—that merely being in her room for what they called a conversation was the kind of human experience that no young doctor should miss. I spoke to Janice about the students' visits before I began making them. She not only agreed, but said that there was a message she wanted to be sure was transmitted to them.

By that time Janice was quadriplegic with flexion contractures at every joint, so that the actual space she occupied in the bed was very small. Because her facial muscles were paralyzed, she could not talk; she was fed via a tube inserted directly into her stomach. In fact, her only motor unit that worked was the frontalis, or forehead muscle, on her right side. One of the engineers had fitted the muscle with an interfacing wire that allowed a kind of Morse-code connection to a bedside computer.

Each time Janice's bed was wheeled into the conference room, I would (of course, this was all with her permission) ask the students whether they'd want to be kept alive, were they in her condition. Before anyone could respond I would ask a student to put the question to Janice directly, and ask her how she felt about being kept going day after day in this state. She always gave the same answer, laboriously and taking what seemed an infinite amount of time, during which I never once saw a student so much as turn his or her eyes away from that computer screen. Here follows Janice's answer:

> *My life may look dehumanized and infantilized, and it is. But I have a window next to my bed, and every morning I watch the sun rise, and hear the birds sing. And for me, that is a gift. That is why, yes, I want to live.*

MY SECOND TALE IS of an entirely different nature—in fact, I've added it for my own sake. One of my titles is director of the Center for Neuroscience and Regeneration Research. Thoughts of regeneration have sweetened the dreams of many a scientist in recent years, especially as the notion of functional stem cells seems to be coming ever closer to reality. From a time in the recent past when talk of the appearance of new neurons or nerve fibers was nothing more than an opportunity to use the word "chimerical" to today's optimism based on stem cell research seems like an eyeblink, and it is. But this present Tale is of a regeneration of quite another sort. It might be said that it is a story in which a bit of pathology re-creates the image of a love no longer physically near, and yet available specifically because something has gone wrong.

Kate and Walter Meuller met at a USO party for returning veterans of the Korean War. Both were shy, and each had
come at the urging of friends. They fell into conversation
that evening only because they were part of a group of eight
or nine young people telling humorous—and some not so
humorous—stories about their boring jobs. Kate chimed in
by pointing out that she thought she must be setting a record
for nonachievement at AT&T, where she had been working
as a stenographer for four years, with no promotion in sight.
Walter thought that was particularly funny, because it approximated his situation in the field artillery. In fact, the party took
place on the very anniversary of his promotion to private first
class four years earlier, a level at which he would remain, he
supposed, until his discharge.

By the time that discharge took place, six months later, Kate
and Walter were engaged. They had begun to date for no particular reason, and decided after a while that wanting constantly
to be together must mean that they were in love. They were
married within a year, and the rest of their lives together was
as easy and unplanned as their meeting and falling in love: no
major triumphs and no major defeats; two children, one of each
kind; a small house in a suburb of Portland, Maine where they
had first met; the usual payments on the usual debts; and all of
the other trimmings that come attached to the usual middle-
class life when the husband is the floor manager of a department
store and the wife is a—well, a wife and a mother. Their son,
George, became a corporal in the field artillery and returned
from Viet Nam at twenty to spend his career as a draughtsman,

and their daughter, Jean, married a fine young man she had met at the same kind of USO party that had ultimately been responsible for her own existence. Like Kate, she became a—well, a wife and a mother. The image I am trying to convey here is of complete ordinariness for this couple, who seemed to epitomize one of the many versions of a particular kind of American dream, enwrapped in contentment and aspiring to good health and love within the normative parameters as we define them.

And this is precisely, as I understand it, what the Meullers had, with one outstanding characteristic that is as much a part of the entire package as everything else within it. By this I mean that they were fortunate enough to never lose that feeling of always wanting to be together. Whereas they had originally seen this as the basis of their love, the passage of years made it only one component of this relationship for which we all, as human beings, seek.

But such happinesses, like life itself, are finite. Without any premonitory signs, eighty-year-old Kate Meuller died of a massive cerebral hemorrhage one summer afternoon while working in her garden. I need not describe the effect on Walter. For months he would speak about nothing but Kate, and stare for hours at every photograph he could find of the two of them together. To no one's surprise, he had only three or four photos of her in which he was not at her side. After all, these were the people who had wanted always to be together, and that fact was reflected in all their recorded memories.

I first met Walter almost a year after Kate's death. About two weeks earlier he had sustained what is known as a transient ischemic attack (or TIA), defined as a strokelike episode lasting less than twenty-four hours. Though fully recovered, he had begun three days later to experience daily well-formed hallucinations, always exactly the same in nature: They were of Kate's face. I recommended that he take a drug called perphenazine, which virtually guarantees that the hallucinations will stop. Can it be a surprise to anyone reading this Tale that he refused to take the drug? "I'd rather see my Kate," he said.

The Urologist's Tale

COMPLEX OPERATIONS PERFORMED BY teams of surgeons are so common nowadays that medical interns and the general public often forget how recently such procedures were not only unusual, but in many ways resembled human experimentation each time they were undertaken. In fact, had we in place some of the highly refined standards of modern bioethics, certain operations might well have undergone delays in their development by as much as years. The other side of the coin, of course, is that we are today properly prevented from certain courses of action by committees of our peers, without whom we might otherwise rush into attempts not justified by the state of technology, the condition of the patient, or our own lack of expertise.

Though some of the early cardiac operations of the 1940s, for example, saved lives that might otherwise have been lost, others were done prematurely, either because the patient seemed so sick or the surgical team felt themselves to be at a more effective state of readiness than was actually the case. When Christian Barnard accomplished the first technically successful cardiac transplantation in December 1967, on a patient named Louis Washkansky, the problems of organ rejection had not yet been solved. Surgeons in England, Canada, Brazil, Argentina, France, and several centers in the United States rushed to duplicate Barnard's feat almost immediately, not realizing that much immunological research still needed to be done. The result was that within fifteen months, 118 operations were performed in eighteen different countries, with the majority of patients dying within weeks or months. A long moratorium was necessary before the notion of cardiac transplantation could be revived by advances in the laboratory, to become the routine procedure with excellent results it is today.

I was involved in one of the early transplantations of a kidney. The problems of rejection had been worked out at the Peter Brent Brigham Hospital in Boston by several researchers, using two drugs called 6-mercaptopurine and a closely related compound called azathioprine. It was not long before effective technical procedures had been developed, and the Boston team performed the first successful kidney transplantation from a cadaver in 1962. Encouraged by the good results, several other centers, notably in Richmond, Virginia, and Denver, Colorado, soon began their own small programs, as did some in a few European countries. Nevertheless, it would be years before there were enough such hospitals and trained personnel prepared for the increasing needs, which remained poorly served for years. Due to an artificial kidney machine having been developed to keep the blood clear of impurities—a process called dialysis—patients were usually enabled to wait until a proper donor became available. But by 1967, when my first patient presented himself, there were still few hospitals where the operation was being done, though many men and women were undergoing frequent dialysis. Using dogs, my team and I had worked out the surgical technique to perfection, and were only awaiting our first patient.

Knowing of our work, Igor Gronski insisted on becoming that first patient. Gronski was a fifty-one-year-old Polish immigrant who had served as a fighter pilot in the Royal Air Force during World War II, and he seemed to fear nothing. Nothing, that is, except the necessity of staying on the restricted diet our nephrologists had prescribed for him while he was on the kidney machine. Having grown up on foods like pickled herring, he was prone to dietary indiscretions and frequently overloaded with salt and water, regardless of our valiant attempts to keep him properly dialyzed. As he himself pointed out, he was holding the equivalent of a gun to our heads, demanding that we go forward at the first opportunity.

Not surprisingly, that first opportunity took place under tragic circumstances. On an overcast day in December 1967, three Canterbury juniors were traveling south on the local interstate when the driver's vision was obscured by smoke from an incinerator and he lost control of his car. Though two of the boys survived with minimal damage, one sustained a severe head injury, was declared brain dead, and was placed on a respirator. His uncle, a physician, immediately notified the boy's parents in California and took the initiative of suggesting that one of the kidneys be used for transplantation. In spite of their grief, or perhaps because of it, they agreed.

Our team began its preparations, and Gronski was immediately notified to come into the hospital. Though I had already told him several times that I had never witnessed a kidney transplant in a human being, I repeated the information again to be absolutely sure he knew what he was letting himself in for. He responded with the enthusiasm we expected, and was brought into one of the operating rooms while several of my staff prepared to remove the donor kidneys in an adjoining recovery room. Just at that moment, I received an agitated phone call from John Stanton, then the director of the hospital, wanting to know why I was doing this procedure without his express permission. I was infuriated that he would dare interfere, and told him so. I had already been given permission to go ahead by Jim Corson, the newly appointed chief of surgery. Emboldened by the fact that Jim was planning to assist me to provide moral support, I hung up on the director and went directly to the small recovery room, where the kidneys had been removed and their vessels and tubules were being rinsed with appropriate biochemical solutions. I stepped into the OR with one of the kidneys in a basin.

The procedure went remarkably well. Within about twenty minutes, I had attached the donor artery and vein to those of the recipient, and was gratified to see the first bit of urine dripping from the ureter, the tubule I was about to connect to Gronski's bladder. Feeling rather proud of myself, I prepared to insert the first stitches when I realized to my horror that I had put the kidney in place upside down. But I suddenly recalled something I had learned in physiology class decades earlier as a first-year medical student: Even a man standing on his head propels urine in the right direction, because the wavelike movement called peristalsis pushes it forward that way. Immensely relieved, I completed the attachment, and was gratified to note that Gronski was continuing to make the first urine he had produced in months. The operation was a complete success. Canterbury was the first American hospital outside of Boston, Richmond, and Denver to have transplanted a kidney.

After about a year and a half, Gronski decided to return home to live in his native Poland, where he was regarded with awe as a miracle of modern medicine. Cortisone preparations were being used at that time to help prevent rejection, but no one, even in the United States, had yet reached the point of standardizing the doses required. One day a few months after his return, I received a telephone call from the urologist who had been treating our patient in Gdansk. Gronski had suddenly developed peritonitis, almost certainly because his rectal wall had been thinned and finally perforated by overdoses of the cortisone. He died within days, a victim of the very progress that had improved his life for almost two years.

૭ર

Commentary to The Urologist's Tale

Igor Gronski was a chimera, just as is every person who carries a transplanted part of another within him. The word "chimera" appears first in Homer's *Iliad,* where it is used to describe a mythical creature that is "a thing of immortal make, not human, lion-fronted and snake behind, a goat in the middle, and snorting out the breath of the terrible flame of bright fire." From this origin comes the modern word, used to signify an idea that is, also like the chimera, fanciful and absurd, in the sense of being impossible to achieve.

By solving the riddle of transplantation, scientists have proven that the chimerical may not be so chimerical after all. Fully formed complex organs are being grafted from one human being to another. We are living in an era in which transplantations are commonly being done of any number of organs, of which the kidney was first.

The story of transplantation is the story of scientists' evolving comprehension that the cells of each of us harbor within them something that is theirs alone, which gives them their unique unchanging character. For want of a better term, we might well call that something by the name "selfness." Once the existence of selfness was appreciated, it became necessary to hunt down its ingredients—what is the specific quality that a cell shares with all of its mates, that makes it so singularly a part of one individual and foreign to all others? What is the mechanism by which an animal recognizes cells that originate in another animal, and what is the mechanism by which it rejects them, destroying them as invading undesirables? And, having discovered the nature of these mechanisms, how may they be overcome?

Graft rejection was gradually recognized as a process similar to the one in which the body produces proteins called antibodies to destroy foreign materials called antigens, such as bacteria. The fluids and cells of the host recognize foreignness and create the substances that lead to its destruction. The search for the major transplantation antigens began in the late 1940s, and by the early 1950s it was possible to carry out a kind of primitive tissue-typing, analogous to the way a pint of blood is typed and cross-matched to a particular recipient.

While tissue-typing is nowadays a much more sophisticated process than it was during the early stages of its development, perfect compatibility will probably never be achieved, since so many minor antigens are involved in the outcome. But two logical avenues have been pursued: making the immune system of the host more tolerant to the transplantation antigens of the donor, and making the donor tissue less menacing. The former approach has been more successful, and proved to be a practical basis on which to carry out continuing research. It is, in fact, the principle upon which present-day transplantation techniques have been developed.

At present, the only situation presenting no immunological problem occurs when the donor and recipient are identical twins, since, coming from the same egg, they have the same antigen. Indeed, the first long-term successful kidney transplant was accomplished between such twins at Boston's Peter Brent Brigham Hospital in 1954.

When it became possible for suppression of the immune system to reach a stage where it was of practical use, the era of clinical organ transplantation began. In October 1953, Peter Medawar and two colleagues published a paper in the journal *Nature* in which they described producing "actively acquired tolerance" by inoculation of mouse cells into another mouse while it was still in utero and had not yet developed its immunological defenses. That this was possible produced a new optimism among researchers, and a great race began to develop the proper drugs to suppress the immune system and the proper criteria for their use. Thus the search for drug-induced tolerance began. Working with one of the surgeons who had done the original twin transplant, Joseph Murray, Roy Calne prepared protocols with the drug 6-mercaptopurine and later the closely related compound azathioprine. The Brigham team achieved such success that it was not long before safe and effective methods of kidney transplantation had been developed in enough American and European centers that the procedure became practical for increasing numbers of recipients. With the use of an artificial kidney machine to clear the blood of impurities, patients were enabled to wait until a proper donor was available, and then to undergo the procedure.

In the majority of recipients, the donor has been a young person just pronounced dead. With proper matching and careful management of immunosuppresion, the so-called cadaver kidney has succeeded more than 80 percent of the time. Other major factors have also been important, such as the use of steroids and the development of cyclosporine, a fungus-derived agent discovered almost by accident in Norway. Cyclosporine has rapidly become the major drug utilized in transplantation. In fact it is fair to say that its introduction has brought such safety to immunosuppression that the figure of more than 80 percent success is largely due to its addition. Though cyclosporine was not available in 1967, when Gronski had his transplant, our urologist used the other drugs, along with steroids, for immunosuppression. The doses of steroid were difficult to manage, and it was for this reason that Gronski eventually died. It is safe to say that, had this remarkable drug been in use at that time, the hero of this story might well still be alive, enjoying his pickled herring at a sidewalk café in Gdansk.

॰

The Pediatrician's Tale

HERE ARE TWO GOOD reasons that this is a short Tale. The first is simply that it has to do with hydrocephalus, and the Narrator tells me that he already has described a patient with this abnormality. But that doesn't stop me, because he also asked me to tell him about the most memorable patient I've ever seen. It happens that the child who fulfills this qualification had hydrocephalus, so he's stuck with the story unless he just wants to discard it. If he decides to keep it, what he gets is a shorter Tale, since I don't have to go into great detail about the disease itself because readers are familiar with it from The Neurosurgeon's Tale(s).

But at least as important a reason for this Tale's brevity has to do with its teller. I'm from Vermont, and we Green Mountain boys are notorious for our reticence: Remember Calvin Coolidge? Hardly said a word in four years in the White House. We're all just like that, so here I go with what I promise is the shortest chapter in this book.

Before joining a group in Boston, I was in solo practice in a small town in my home state for about ten years. Now, a small town by Vermont standards is really small—the whole state has only half a million people in it. So you can imagine that when a family moves here from a city as big as Buffalo, there are some things they have to get used to. The family I'm writing about had a four-year-old boy with congenital hydrocephalus, and they suddenly found their little fellow being cared for by a hick pediatrician—me, of course—instead of the professor of neurosurgery who had been following him since he was born. The mother, about as nervous a woman as I've ever known, had been told that the hydrocephalus had been "arrested," whatever that means, and had therefore not required a shunt. She was told to bring the boy back for follow-up every three months, at which time the professor would measure his head with a simple tape measure, ask a few questions about his development, scrawl a sentence or two in his chart, and make the next appointment. My guess is that he thought this well-meant frequent follow-up would reassure the mom, but it turned out to have the opposite effect.

The first time I saw the boy, he seemed perfectly normal except for a minimally increased head size. The child worried me a lot less than his mother, who was the proverbial "basket case" with concern about whether the hydrocephalus was insidiously progressing, and causing as-yet undetectable brain damage. She had never been quite comfortable with the professor's care, having expected all kinds of complex surgery yet seeing her child being examined with nothing more sophisticated than the tape measure. She treated the boy as if he needed to be watched every second for fear that something awful would happen if she took her eye off him even momentarily. Reassurance by a Buffalo psychiatrist had been of no help, and he finally put her on some kind of tranquilizer. Meantime, the Buffalo neurosurgeon had retired, and she knew nothing about the incoming chief.

One of the nicest things about practicing in a very small town is that things never get busy, so doctors can spend as much time as they want to with each patient. Of course, this is especially true in a state like Vermont, where nothing ever moves very quickly anyway. So I had plenty of time to talk to Mrs. Hurlburt, whose nervousness made her far more voluble than all but a few mothers in my small practice. After a long conversation, it finally became clear to me that she was struggling with the seeming contradiction between a condition about which the word "arrested" is used and the necessity for frequent follow-ups and measurements, albeit of such a basic kind.

I thought a great deal about the uncertainty principle that afternoon and decided to take the bull by the horns. I told the mom that the frequent visits could stop, measurements would be taken only at the child's regular checkups, and that I felt confident that too much attention was being paid to the little fellow. I called the new chief of neurosurgery in Buffalo and told him what I was doing. Though reluctant to change his predecessor's plan, he agreed to agree.

I saw the boy regularly during my remaining five years in the small town, measured his head only on every other visit, and Mom stopped taking the pills. She wrote to me in Boston on his twenty-first birthday, to tell me that he was fine and a junior at the University of Vermont. No one had measured his head in years.

The Narrator's Tale

I N A BOOK DEVOTED, at least partially, to "the most memorable patient I've ever known," there should certainly be a few pages devoted to "the most memorable *doctor* I've ever known," or perhaps "the most memorable doctor experience I've ever heard of." And so, I'll take what I call Narrator's Privilege—if there is such a thing—and tell the story of a man born in a small room above a grocery store in Brooklyn who rose to become one of the major figures in American medicine, in an adventure-filled life of eighty-seven years. The most exciting of the adventures is the one recorded here.

Danny Farber kept the light of much of his professional life so well hidden under a bushel that I had to uncover a considerable portion of the Tale you are about to read while speaking at various times to mutual friends and professional colleagues. He had a way of becoming completely frank about matters never previously discussed, so he was not reluctant to confirm details as I questioned him after turning up some particularly interesting bit of biography. The interesting bit of biography I'm about to relate here is, by my lights, the most fascinating interval in a life filled with fascinations.

Danny's story actually does begin in the tiny family apartment in which both he and his younger brother, Al, were born in the years just before the United States entered World War I. Both excelled academically in high school and matriculated at Columbia College on scholarships. Danny would have loved to go on to the College of Physicians and Surgeons at Columbia, but those were the days of tight ethnic quotas, so his medical degree was obtained at New York University and Bellevue Hospital. He took an internship and residency in internal medicine, and was surprised to find himself interested in anesthesiology, a specialty then so poorly regarded that even the presence of the famous Dr. E. A. Rovenstine on that small faculty attracted few residents to the field.

But history had other plans for Danny. Within a year of Pearl Harbor, he enlisted as a medical officer in what was then called the Army Air Force, and he served at several military hospitals before being assigned to a large base in England, from which American planes left every day for huge bombing raids over Germany. His job was to attend to wounded crew members as the aircraft returned, and he had plenty of trauma experience by the time he had been at those duties for six months. Because there was no formal name for what he was doing, he did not realize that he was also learning—and inventing as he worked on these young men—the basics of resuscitation and the management of fluid and blood replacement after major trauma, skills that would prove so important as he later developed the field of physiology-based anesthesia.

Danny was a meticulous observer, and the thought came to him that he would understand trauma and fluid balance far better if he could only see how the wounds were sustained. He began to harangue one of his pilot friends to take him on a mission or two, but there were strict rules against such things. Still, Danny persisted, and one day his friend consented to bring him on a raid over Strasbourg, considered to be safe enough and short enough that the likelihood of being shot down was remote, though there might be some injuries caused by the jolting effect of German anti-aircraft. The raid itself was exactly as planned and expected, the payload was dropped, and the unscathed B-17 was soon on its way home, with Danny having made some significant observations during the actively evasive portion of the run. Unfortunately, the aircraft was hit by flack as it was returning over Vichy France.

When it became obvious that the plane was going down, the pilot handed Danny a parachute, strapped him into it, showed him the ripcord, and told him to jump. Danny would later tell me that he has no recollection of whether he did or

did not have time to do as he was told, but only that he awak-
ened two days later, lying on a stretcher with his left arm and
chest heavily bandaged and being conveyed by four members
of the French resistance toward the Pyrenees. He never had any
idea what had happened during those two days, but soon was
informed that he and one of the crew were the only survivors
of the crash. Once the resistance men had gotten him and the
other American into Spain, they were quickly transported via
ambulance to a military hospital (late in the war, Franco seems
to have been hospitable to allied soldiers), where Danny's broken left arm and clavicle were treated. Not until he returned
to the States three weeks later did he find out that the blunt
injury to his chest was so severe that a huge rent had been torn
in his diaphragm. He would spend almost the rest of his life
with a portion of his stomach upside down and adherent to his
left lung, a problem that required careful dietary management
because he repeatedly refused surgery until it underwent torsion
when he was eighty-four years old, necessitating a difficult and
very hazardous emergency procedure.

A few weeks after September 11, 2001, I noticed a medal in
Danny's lapel of which I had no previous knowledge. He made
light of my question concerning its provenance, saying that he
was wearing it only because "all these old World War II fogies
have suddenly trotted out their European and Asian Theater
combat medals, so I decided to wear this to be one up." It was
the Silver Star, our nation's third highest military award for heroism in combat. Though Danny denied remembering the words
of the citation, I later found out that it was awarded for acts of

heroism of which he has no memory, carried out after the B-17 crashed and before he lost consciousness. They must have been reported by the other survivor. Not only had Danny saved that man's life, but he was tending to the injuries of several others when the resistance appeared.

Danny's medical discharge in early 1945 was followed by his return to Bellevue to complete a full residency with Rovenstine in anesthesiology. By then he had witnessed not only the importance of proper blood and fluid balance but also the sparsity of qualified physicians in the field. Rovenstine arranged for him to be hired by the Columbia group, but he refused to take the job unless he was made chief, since he was the only fully trained man on the staff. Not only did he insist on being chief, but he made the further demand that anesthesiology become a completely separate and independent department. The university had little choice, even though all other such units were within departments of surgery except those at Oxford, the University of Wisconsin, and NYU. Though they did it figuratively kicking and screaming, Columbia thus acquired a new department, and a new thirty-five-year-old chairman fully trained in internal medicine. The year was 1952.

Danny immediately set about utilizing all he knew of such matters as kidney and cardiac function to supplement his hard-won knowledge of fluid management and major trauma. Being able to attract a group of highly motivated young residents added to the luster of his new department, and before long there were many research papers coming out of it. His reputation soared. As new departments of anesthesia were being created in the 1950s and 1960s, his became one of the most sought-after and competitive. With some five or six other chairmen and unit directors, Danny Farber transformed his specialty, which is why the History of Anesthesia Society lists him among a small group to whom they refer as The Legends of Anesthesia.

Danny spent twenty-five years at Columbia, turning down several offers to become dean of one or another medical school. He had a motive, which was to take a school of not very well-respected quality and do with it what he had done with his own specialty: turn it into something recognized as being of high caliber. In this, too, he succeeded, at the University of Florida.

There is a great deal more to tell about Danny Farber, including his multiple prizes for scientific achievement; special government missions all over Europe and Asia; honorary degrees and other awards from foreign nations; and finally the degree for which he worked so hard after retiring as dean at Florida after fourteen years: a Ph.D. in English Literature, which he attained at age seventy-six by completing his doctoral thesis on the topic he later published in the form of a remarkable book entitled *Romance, Poetry and Surgical Sleep: Literature Influences Medicine*.

It would be unfair both to Danny and to his intriguing thesis were I to attempt summarizing the argument of his dissertation, but the basic point he makes is that the Romantic Movement in literature and poetry altered society's views about pain and suffering. Once this occurred, methods of inducing analgesia and surgical sleep—which had barely changed in millennia—became important objects of research, resulting in the use of such agents as sulfuric ether and nitrous oxide in the mid-1840s. Both of these agents had been well known (ether for almost three hundred years), but not until the vast cultural concern for one another's suffering eventuated during the Romantic period did it seem of significance to do anything about what were previously considered the natural consequences of being a human being on this planet.

Even Danny's death was unique. Determined to understand the intricacies of Islamic thought after the attacks of September 11, 2001, he devoted a great deal of time to studying the religion and its associated worldview, and at one point organized a conference with that theme at the Aspen Institute, where he had for many years been on the board of directors. Late one afternoon during early December 2002, he was seeking new information on the Internet when he complained of a sudden blurring of vision and fell to the floor. Five hours later, he was dead of a cerebral hemorrhage at the age of eighty-seven.

Danny's was a well-lived life, filled with the joy of hard work, the love of family and groups of interesting friends, and the rewards of the many contributions he made to science and to the comfort and accomplishments of others. He was, indeed, the most memorable doctor I've ever known. What I have recorded here is the merest hint of what he did, and what he meant to those of us fortunate enough to have had close relationships with him. Though surgical sleep will remain always the professional heritage with which he is associated, it was his poetry and romance for which we remember him most.

Epilogue

WE HAVE READ HERE of unusual diseases, such as hydrocephalus, seen every day by certain specialists; and of common diseases, such as diabetes, that can devastate a person's life by certain of their manifestations. We have read of seemingly minor problems, as in The Dermatologist's Tale, that cause misery far out of proportion to their actual effect on the body, and of diseases so devastating that they threaten life, and yet go on to what would seem a spontaneous cure. A twentieth-century case is described that harkens back to a problem that killed a man four hundred years earlier, and other patients are beset with diseases unrecognized or untreatable

until the recent past. We have read of transactions between doctor and patient that changed the life of each forever, and of
transactions that barely extended beyond the period of diagnosis and therapy. In virtually every situation, the patient is the
teacher of the doctor, though neither may realize it at the time.
In every case, we see a candid photo of this peculiar kinship that
has come to be called the doctor-patient relationship, whether
it seems superficial, as in The Surgeon's Tale, or profound, as in
the tales of the Cardiologist and Internist. As has been said of
the history of medicine itself, all of life is there. Each doctor is,
knowingly or not, a philosopher.

Most of the stories in this book are told by physicians near
or past the end of their careers, so they combine to provide an
image of medicine as it has been practiced over the course of
the past half-century. Their topics range from the treatment of
a bleeding polyp to organ transplantation, from simple observation of an abnormal structure to technologies that approach
the most advanced that medicine now offers. But by and large,
they deal with a period that drew to a close in the 1970s, when
the bionic wonders of ultramodern medicine began gradually to
replace the hands-on methods that had drawn so many thoughtful young people into the profession. This is not to say that today's
young physicians are not as thoughtful as their predecessors—it
is simply to point out that the powerful diagnostic tools of the
twenty-first century have largely replaced the more meticulous
considerations of the signs and symptoms of the average patient.
Physical examination and history-taking are still the origins of
diagnosis, but seem not as important as they were only thirty

years ago, because some large, expensive machine will reveal what might have been missed by the old methods.

For the most part, all of this is to the good, because diagnosis is today swifter and more accurate (though much more expensive) than it was in the past, as is therapy. But something has been lost, and it is impossible to tell whether the loss is important or not. The ultimate mainstay of diagnosis is not data, information, or even knowledge—it is judgment. Are the advantages of being able to obtain so much data being lost by the disadvantages of categorizing patients or of thinking algorithmically about diagnosis and therapy? The medical schools have recognized this problem, and they provide courses in clinical judgment. As Hippocrates told his colleagues almost two and a half millennia ago, judgment will always be the most difficult aspect of the art of medicine.

Index

A

Abdominal pain, 129–30
Advance directives, 61–62
Air Force Medical School, 50
Allopathic medicine, 32
American Cancer Society, 27
American College of
    Physicians, 152
American College of Surgeons, 116
Amyotrophic lateral sclerosis,
    176–78
*Anatomy of the Bronchopulmonary
    Segments,* 138
Anemia, 149

Anesthesiologist, 73–85
Anesthesiology, 201–2
Ankle joint pain, 124–25, 130–31
Anticancer drugs, 126
Antihistamines, 32
Antilymphocytic globulin, 169
Appendicitis, 133–34
Army Air Force, 198
Arthritis, 124–25
Aseptic meningitis, 147–51
Aspen Institute, 203
Atypical pneumonia, 149
Auschwitz, 36–37
Autopsy, 132, 146

Ayres, Lew, 17
Azathioprine, 184, 190

B
B&O Railroad, 173
Baby delivery, 43
Balantidium, 148
Balloon pump, 56, 60
Barker, Lewellys, 153
Barnard, Christian, 184
Behcet, Hulusi, 125–26
Behcet's disease, 125–34
Bellevue Hospital, 198, 201
Berry, General Frank, 45–46
Bioethics, 60–61, 63, 79–85.
    See related Ethics
Bipolar disorder, 82–83
Blade cut, 6–7
Blastocystis, 148
Breast
    Biopsy of, 20–21
    cancer, axilla lymph nodal
        spread, 22–25
    lump in, 18
Breech delivery, 51–52, 54
Bronchoscope, 136–38
Bronchoscopist, 135–42

C
Canterbury Tales, x
Cardiac rhythm disturbance, 57
Cardiac transplantation, 170, 184
Cardiologist, 55–63, 206
Carina, 137
Cerebral hemorrhage, 180, 203
Cervix, 42–43
Cesarean section, 91

Chaucer, Geoffrey, x
Chemotherapy, 25, 29
Chest surgeon, 101–16
Child abuse, 87–90
Chimera, 188
Cholecystectomy, 79–85
Clubbing (finger tips), 125–26
Colicky pain, 7, 10
Colon
    cancer, 39
    perforation, 5–6
    reattachment, 14
Colonoscopy, 39
Columbia College, 198, 201–2
Computerized tomography scan,
    125, 130
Confidentiality, x
Congenital diaphragmatic
    hernias, 6
Congestive heart failure, 55–63,
    170
Contact dermatitis, 33
Coolidge, Calvin, 194
Cordus, Valerius, 13
Coronary artery bypass grafts,
    56, 60
Coronary artery disease, 170
Cortisone, 32, 126, 187–88
CPB (cocamidopropyl), 33
Crying, 161–71
Cushing, Harvey, 94, 95, 96, 97
Cyclosporine, 126, 191

D
D'Alon, Captain François,
    10–11, 12
Dakin's chloride solution, 121

Decision-making, 38–39
Defibrillator, 57, 60
Dehydration, 129–30
Dermatitis, 33
Dermatologist, 31–33, 205
Diabetes, 162–74, 205
    neuropathy in, 166
    retinopathy in, 165, 169
Dialysis, 170, 185
Diaphragm, 4–5
Dislocated shoulder, 156–57
DMAPA (dimethylamino-
    proylamine), 33
"Doctor Himself as Therapeutic
    Agent, The," 152–53
Doctor-patient relationships,
    ix, xi, 206. *See also specific
    specialists*
Ductus arteriosus, 68, 103–5,
    110–11
Durable Power of Attorney, 61

E
Electrocardiogram, 171
Emergency room, 129–31
English Literature, 202
Ether, 13, 84, 202
    -induced sleep, 12–13
Ethics, x, xi, 74–75.
    See related Bioethics
Euthanasia, 60

F
Family physician, 17–30
Farber, Danny, 197–203
Feculent empyema, 2, 5, 6,
    11–12, 156

Finger amputation, 136
Food and Drug Administration,
    128
Ford, Betty, 26
Foreign body removal, child's
    lung, 139–42
Francis, Arlene, 17
Futile treatment, 61–62

G
Galen, 143–45, 147, 150–51,
    153
Gallbladder surgery, 79–85
Gastroenterologist, 35–30
Genital cellulitis, 117–22
Genital ulcers, 126
Geriatric patient, 38
Geriatrician, 123–34
Graft rejection, 189
Gutenberg Bible, 55

H
Hallucinations, 181
Harvard, 13
Head measurements, 195–96
Health Care Proxy, 61
Heart attack, 56
Hematoma, 157–59
Hemorrhagic stroke, 170
Hippocrates, 36, 124, 131,
    153–54, 207
Hippocratic Oath, 74
History of Anesthesia Society, 202
History-taking, 133, 206–7
Holocaust survivors, 35–36
Homer, 188
Hopkins, Mr., 172–74

Hormone treatment, 25
Houston, W. S., 152–53
Human lessons, ix
Hydrocephalus, 90–99, 194–96, 205
Hymen, 19–20
Hymenotomy, 21, 23, 30

I
Iliad, 188
Immunosuppression, 169, 190–91
Impaired surgeon, 77–78, 80–85
Internist, 143–54, 206
Islam, 203
Italian night whorehouse, 117–22

J
Jaundice, 149
Johns Hopkins Medical School, 94, 153, 172–74
Judgment, 207

K
Kidney
    failure, 170
    transplantation, 184–88
Korean War, 179

L
Laennec, René, 132
Legends of Anesthesia, 202
Living, 177–78
Long, Crawford, 13
Lou Gehrig's disease, 176–78
Lung
    cancer, 125–26, 130–31
    collapse, 13

M
Magnetic resonance imaging (MRI) scans, 27
Malpractice, 73–85
Mammogram, 25, 27
Marital love story, 179–81
Massachusetts General Hospital, 12–13, 84
Mastectomy, 20–23, 25–26, 29
Measles, 148
Medical ethics. *See* Bioethics, Ethics
Medical student, 117–22
Meigs, Charles de Lucena, 162
Memoirs, 59–60
Memorial Sloan-Kettering Hospital, 26
Meningitis, 147–51
Mentor-student relationship, xi
Merthiolate, 21, 141
Military medical needs, 45–54
Misbehavior, 104–5
Morgagni, Giovanni, 132
Morpheus, 84
Morphine, 42
Muscle aches, 149
Myocarditis, 149

N
Narrator, 197–203
Nephrologist, 161–74
Neurologist, 175–81
Neurosurgeon, 87–99
New York University, 198, 201
Nitrous oxide, 202
Nobel Prize in Medicine, 26
Nursing homes, 123

O

Obstetrician-gynecologist, 41–43
On Mediate Auscultation, 132
Operative permit, 3, 20–21
Ophthalmologist, 45–54
Oral ulcers, 126
Osteoarthritis, 36
Oxford, 201

P

Pancreas transplant, 163–70
Paré, Ambroise, 9–11, 12, 14
Parks, Rosa, 48
Pasteur, Louis, 147
Pastoral care, 62–63
Patch tests, 33
Patent ductus arteriosus.
    See Ductus arteriosus
Pathology, frozen specimen, 21–22
Patient
    confidence, 147–54
    -doctor relationship, ix, xi, 206.
    See also specific specialists
    individuality, 37
Patient Self-Determination
    Act of 1990, 61
Pearl Harbor, 198
Pediatric cardiologist, 65–72
Pediatric neurosurgery, 87–99
Pediatrician, 193–96
Pelvic exam, 18–19
Penicillin, 121
Peristalsis, 185
Peritonitis, 51, 187–88
Perphenazine, 181
Physical examination, 131–34,
    206–7

Physician-assisted suicide, 60
Physiology-based anesthesia,
    199
Pneumonia, 13, 149
Pregnancy, 51–52
Prescription, 58–59
Prostatic cancer, 130
Pulmonary stenosis, 69

R

Racism, 48–50, 53–54
Radiation, 25, 29
Rash, upper eyelid, 32–33
Rectal tear, 88
Regeneration, 178
Remote superiority attitude,
    93, 94–96, 97
Respirator, 170–71
Rockefeller, Happy, 26
*Romance, Poetry and Surgical
    Sleep: Literature Influences
    Medicine,* 202
Romantic Movement, 202–3
Rovenstine, E. A., 198, 201
Royal Air Force, 185

S

Scoundrel, 110–16
Selfness, 188–89
Shampoo, 33
Shunts, 92, 98, 99
Sigmoidoscopy, 37–38
Silver Star, 200–201
6-mercaptopurine, 184, 190
Skin ulcers, 126
Splenectomy, 157–59
Sporotrichosis, 148

Stethoscope, 132
Stillbirth, 52
Stomach torsion, 200
Street kid, 1–15
Strep throat, 148
Streptomycin, 121
Sulfuric ether, 202.
    See related Ether
Surgeon, 155–59, 206
Surgery, 1–15
Surgical anesthesia, 12–13
Surgical chief, 8–9
Surgical quirks, 66–72
Surgical sleep, 202–3.
    See also Anesthesia

T
Tetracycline, 121
Thalidomide, 127–28
Thoracic surgeons, 137–38
Thoracotomy, 141–42
Tissue typing, 189
Transcient ischemic attack
    (TIA), 180–81
Transplantations, 184–85,
    188–91
Trysts, 107–9, 111

Tuberculosis, 105
Type I diabetes, 162–74.
    See related Diabetes

U
Ulcers, 126
University of Wisconsin, 201
Urologist, 183–91
Uterine contractions, 51

V
Vagina, double, 43
Valvulotome, 70–72
Venable, James, 13
Viet Nam, 179

W
Warren, John Collins, 13
Washkansky, Louis, 184
Water on brain, 90–99
Williams, Esther, 17
Women in medicine, 161–74
Women's movement, 173–74
Works of Ambroise Paré, 9–11
World War I, 198
World War II, 66, 101, 138, 185

ABOUT THE AUTHOR

SHERWIN B. NULAND is Clinical Professor of Surgery at the Yale University School of Medicine, where he also teaches bioethics and medical history, and a Fellow at Yale's Institute for Social and Policy Studies. He is the author of over ten books, including *The Uncertain Art: Thoughts on a Life in Medicine*, *The Art of Aging: A Doctor's Prescription for Well-Being*, and the National Book Award-winning, *How We Die: Reflections on Life's Final Chapter*, a study of the clinical, biological, and emotional details of dying that spent 34 weeks on *The New York Times* best-seller list. Besides being a regular contributor to medical journals, he has written for leading publications such as *The New Yorker, The New Republic*, and *The New York Review of Books*. He lives in Connecticut.

ABOUT THE TYPE

ADOBE GARAMOND is a contemporary typeface family based on the roman types of Claude Garamond and the italic types of Robert Granjon.

Some of the most widely used and influential typefaces in history are those created by the 16th century type designer Claude Garamond. His roman types are arguably the best conceived typefaces ever designed, displaying a superb balance of elegance and practicality.

As Claude Garamond created exceptional roman types, Robert Granjon designed some of the most beautiful italics. Granjon italics have a sloped and energetic look that is both dynamic and practical.

–Excerpted from Adobe's Website (*www.Adobe.com*)